PAPUA NEW GUINEA

Personal Development

Teacher Resource Book

Kenneth Rouse

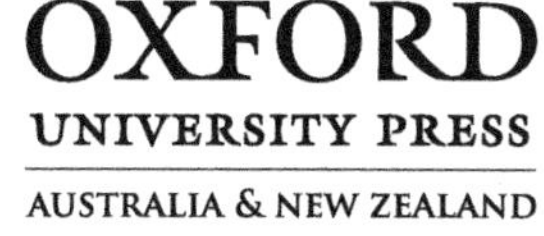

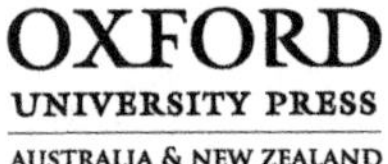

253 Normanby Road, South Melbourne, Victoria 3205, Australia

Oxford University Press is a department of the University of Oxford.
It furthers the University's objective of excellence in research, scholarship, and education by publishing worldwide in

Oxford New York

Auckland Cape Town Dar es Salaam Hong Kong Karachi
Kuala Lumpur Madrid Melbourne Mexico City Nairobi
New Delhi Shanghai Taipei Toronto

With offices in

Argentina Austria Brazil Chile Czech Republic France Greece
Guatemala Hungary Italy Japan Poland Portugal Singapore
South Korea Switzerland Thailand Turkey Ukraine Vietnam

OXFORD is a trademark of Oxford University Press in the UK and in certain other countries

First published 2005
Reprinted 2006, 2007, 2008, 2009, 2010, 2016(D)

ISBN 978 0 19 555881 4

Designed and typeset by Lynn Twelftree
Printed and bound in Australia by Ligare Book Printers Pty Ltd

Contents

Acknowledgements

The Upper Primary Personal Development syllabus was prepared by the Curriculum Development Division of the Department of Education and was coordinated by Colette Modagai.

The publishers would like to acknowledge the assistance of the Curriculum Development Division in the preparation of these resources, in particular Colette Modagai.

These resources were developed with the support of the Australian Government through the Curriculum Reform Implementation Project and the publishers would like to acknowledge the assistance of Dr Graham Dawson, Barbara Hodgins and Mostyn Coleman.

Photo acknowledgements
The authors and publishers wish to thank the following authors and copyright holders for granting permission to reproduce their material:
Corbis/Australian Picture Library: p. 43 (left); AFP/Pool: p. 43 (right).

Secretary's Message

The Upper Primary Personal Development Syllabus is based on the Curriculum Principles of Our Way of Life and Integral Human Development that focus on healthy living, an active lifestyle, pride in our culture, lifestyles and values, the importance of relationships, and living and working together harmoniously. Students will play an informed role in both individual and community actions that will foster physical, social, emotional, mental and spiritual wellbeing.

This syllabus addresses a wide range of personal, social and community health issues such as reproductive health, growth in population, nutrition, physical activity, safety, HIV and AIDS, drugs and alcohol, the abuse of freedom and rights and peer pressure. Topics of this nature are important issues facing our society today.

Consultation and cooperation between school, home and community will ensure the topics are addressed in a way that supports the role of parents and is sensitive to the values, attitudes, beliefs and practices of the community. All students, both female and male, should be encouraged to participate in all activities to enable them to reach their full potential in all aspects of their lives, and to realise the importance of being a respected, responsible citizen.

Student Books 1 and 2, and the accompanying Teacher Resource Book, have been prepared to provide direct support for the achievement of syllabus outcomes. The content is consistent with, and promotes the teaching and learning models of, the syllabus and the related Department of Education Teachers Guide. These resources encompass a range of material including student activities, advice to teachers, assessment ideas, homework activities, project activities, reference information and a glossary of terms. They are intended to facilitate flexible learning activity for teachers and students, and may be modified and amended to suit local circumstances.

I commend and approve these materials for use in all Upper Primary schools throughout Papua New Guinea.

Peter M. Baki

Peter M. Baki CBE
Secretary for Education

Overview

Personal Development

'Personal Development' is concerned with the holistic development of a person and the focus is to provide opportunities to encourage and support each person in their development. The subject promotes the curriculum principles of Our Way of Life and Integral Human Development. It provides opportunities for students to know how to interact positively with each other and to develop physically, mentally and socially to their fullest potential in order to live productively.

Personal Development addresses health issues that are important to people in Papua New Guinea and gives students the opportunity to develop health care practices to prevent or reduce the risk of illness and disease. Taking part in physical activity is an important part of Personal Development and contributes to healthy living. Personal Development emphasises rules and laws as well as the duties and obligations each citizen has in relation to these laws.

Student books

Key features

The content of the student books is designed to be applicable to the diversity of learning contexts of students in Papua New Guinea. The success of implementing Personal Development depends on the abilities of the teacher to adapt the curriculum and learning materials to the context of the local community. Consequently, the content is flexible in that students in both rural and urban areas can relate to the information. Both the text and the illustrations reflect diverse contexts such as islands, highlands and mainland coastal environments.

The content of these books supports student learning for the Personal Development curriculum area. The books:

- directly support and supplement the upper primary syllabus by following the sequence of strands and sub-strands, with one chapter or section for each strand and clearly identifiable topics for each sub-strand
- contain direct references to the new upper primary syllabus at the beginning of each chapter, demonstrating the clear relationship between the student book and the syllabus
- provide topics and learning approaches that directly support the achievement of syllabus outcomes. The subject content is based on the topics listed under 'Recommended Knowledge' subheadings in the 'Elaborations' section of the *Personal Development Teachers Guide*
- include a wide range of student activities at the end of each topic (which can be completed inside and outside the classroom), reference information and a glossary of terms. Most activities in the 'For You to Try' sections were derived from ideas under 'Recommended Skills and Suggested Activities' in the 'Elaborations' section of the *Personal Development Teachers Guide*

- use icons to indicate where book content has major links to other upper primary subjects
- are written at a reading level that is appropriate for upper primary students and with a format that allows teachers to use it in ways that best suit their objectives and personal teaching style
- draw extensively on examples that are culturally appropriate to upper primary students in Papua New Guinea, giving recognition and credibility to Papua New Guinean knowledge and customs
- use language that is gender sensitive and include positive gender roles
- use text as the main medium of the activity-based approach and include a good proportion of pictures and illustrations to support text
- require only those resources that are normally available to teachers in Papua New Guinea, especially those in rural and remote areas

Teacher Resource Book

Key features

The Teacher Resource Book, in conjunction with the Personal Development student books Book 1 and 2, will help teachers implement the Personal Development syllabus for upper primary students. It provides teachers with the following information:

- relevant information for planning a school-based program
- topics cross-referenced to other curriculum areas to allow for the development of integrated units of work
- a selection of teaching and learning strategies
- ideas for assessment activities
- topic elaborations to show how to develop topics covered in the student books into units of work
- how to extend and develop relevant content and contexts from the student books
- additional information that will assist teachers to develop their own units of work
- additional projects, investigations and activities to further extend students' skills

How to use it

When you receive this book you need to:

- read it carefully to get a sense of the information it contains and how it is organised
- read it carefully to become familiar with the strands and sub-strands, processes and skills, elaborations of learning outcomes and the teaching and learning strategies
- consider how to use the information to develop your own programs and units of work

Structure

The Teacher Resource Book is structured in the following way:

- Each chapter covers one syllabus strand for Personal Development (Strand 1: Relationships, Strand 2: Movement and Physical Activity, Strand 3: Our Culture, Lifestyle and Values, Strand 4: Health of Individuals and Population, Strand 5: Living and Working Together).
- At the beginning of each chapter there is an **overview page** which highlights:
    - ➢ the outcomes of the strand and sub-strands
    - ➢ how these outcomes are developed over the three upper primary grade levels
    - ➢ key words and concepts used and developed throughout the chapter
    - ➢ possible assessment tasks that could be carried out to assess students' knowledge and skills
    - ➢ identified content that has major links to other upper primary subjects

- **Teacher information**—in this section added information is given to that already in the student book to enable teachers to develop units of work. A sample unit is also included at the end of the book to show how a unit of work can be developed over a period of time to achieve specific outcomes.
- The **appendices** at the end of this book include:
  - ➢ projects and investigations from the two student books
  - ➢ a complete glossary
- **Icons**—there are icons throughout the student books. These icons indicate strong links to other subject areas. For example when dealing with preparing food, the icon will be the Personal Development icon to show that food and hygiene are connected.
  The icons look like this:

ML MAL = Making a Living

M M = Mathematics

PD PD = Personal Development

L L = Language

A A = Arts

S S = Science

SS SS = Social Science

Teaching and learning

Outcomes-based education

Outcomes-based education is used in many countries to identify and monitor progress in student learning. A set of outcomes is written to measure the success of teaching a learning unit, topic or course. These outcomes are measurable and can be used to assess if student learning has taken place. An outcomes approach to education means identifying what students should achieve and focusing on ensuring that they do achieve. It means shifting away from an emphasis on what is to be taught and how and when, to an emphasis on what is actually learnt by each student.

The impact of outcomes-based programs on teacher planning and assessment has been significant. Teachers have had to shift from focusing on teaching a subject to focusing on planning for student learning.

Learning Outcomes

The Personal Development syllabus makes explicit the knowledge, skills, attitudes and values that students should achieve in Grades 6, 7 and 8 and are expressed as learning outcomes and indicators. These outcomes describe specifically what students know and are able to do in each strand and grade. The outcomes are broad and can be achieved in any context depending on available resources and expertise. They are student-centred and written in terms that enable them to be demonstrated, assessed and measured.

A student-centred approach focuses on learning as being the active construction of meaning by students, and teaching as the act of guiding and facilitating learning. Examples would include:

- building on students' prior knowledge
- bringing the community and its resources into the school and providing opportunities for students to go out into the community to learn

- providing opportunities for problem-solving, decision-making and taking action
- providing students with opportunities to reflect upon their own learning, knowledge, values, attitudes and skills

Learning outcomes are also developmental, showing progression from one level to the next. For example:

6.5.4 Describe familiar rules and laws of the community, families and schools.

↓

7.5.4 Explain the purpose and benefits of laws in our society.

↓

8.5.4 Describe what duties and obligations people have in upholding society's laws.

Developmental outcomes aim to develop students who are able to:

- reflect and explore a variety of strategies to learn effectively
- participate as responsible citizens in the life of local and national communities
- be culturally sensitive across a range of social contexts
- explore education and career opportunities
- develop income-generating opportunities

Each learning outcome is illustrated with a list of things that students know and can do in order to show that they are achieving an outcome. These are called *indicators*. Indicators are included in a syllabus to help exemplify the range of observable sample behaviours that contribute to the achievement of outcomes linked to the content. They can be used by teachers to monitor student progress within a level and to make judgements about the achievement of an outcome. It is important not to confuse indicators with content.

Learning outcomes and indicators will:

- give teachers the flexibility to develop programs to meet the needs of their students
- help teachers assess and report students' achievements in relation to the learning outcomes
- allow student achievement of the outcomes to be described in consistent ways
- help teachers monitor student learning
- help teachers plan their future teaching programs
- describe what most students will know and be able to do as a result of effective teaching and learning
- help teachers develop student activities for units of work

In summary, outcomes provide a scope and sequence of student learning. They provide a useful focus for planning units of work and report student achievements. Indicators assist in the assessment and reporting process, and in the achievement of learning objectives.

Strategies

The approach to Personal Development is student-centred and provides students with opportunities to practise critical and creative thinking, problem-solving and decision-making. It involves the use of skills and processes such as recall, application, analysis, synthesis, prediction and evaluation, all of which contribute to the development and enhancement of critical thinking. This approach also encourages students to reflect on and monitor their thinking as they make *informed* decisions and take *appropriate* actions.

While working towards their goals, students develop communication skills to enable them to work with others to discuss issues, needs, values, feelings, opinions and attitudes. These skills include:

- interpersonal skills of listening, speaking, responding, being assertive, questioning and justifying a position
- skills in presenting feelings, ideas, views, decisions and findings in written or graphic forms or through movement or drama
- literacy skills such as reading, writing and speaking in ways that suit the context and audience, using the specialised language of Personal Development

There are three possible types of student-centred approach that can be used in Personal Development.

Approach 1: Personal Development process approach

- This approach incorporates all the processes and skills that students will need to develop and use and involves four steps:
  - ➢ gathering information
  - ➢ analysing information
  - ➢ taking action
  - ➢ evaluation and reflection

Approach 2: Inquiry-based approach

- This approach focuses on students developing problem-solving and decision-making skills and skills needed to demonstrate outcomes. This approach involves four phases:
  - ➢ understanding
  - ➢ planning
  - ➢ acting
  - ➢ reflecting

Approach 3: Three-step approach: orienting, enhancing, synthesising (OES)

- There are three phases to this approach:
  - ➢ orientate
  - ➢ enhance
  - ➢ synthesise

More details of each of these three approaches to student-centred learning are found in the *Personal Development Teachers Guide* (pages 5–9). You will need to choose which approach best suits your personal style of teaching and the students in the community in which you are working.

There needs to be a balance between teacher- and student-centred learning. One without the other does not constitute a totally effective teaching approach. Teachers need to:

- choose activities relevant to the students' experiences
- encourage children to tackle problems in their own way
- be flexible in the way students are grouped for different activities
- listen to what students say since this provides valuable insights into their thinking
- encourage students to take risks and to learn from their errors
- recognise links between prior knowledge and new information
- explain, discuss and describe the work they are doing and the ideas they are developing

Students will then be able to:

- identify and solve problems and make decisions using critical and creative thinking
- work effectively with others as members of a team, organisation and community
- organise and manage themselves and their activities responsibly and effectively
- collect, analyse, organise and critically evaluate information
- communicate effectively
- demonstrate an understanding of the world as a set of related systems by recognising that problem-solving contexts do not exist in isolation

Teaching methods

There are three main teaching strategies that can be applied for the learning of new information:

Theory learning (i.e. explicit teaching)—The teacher imparts knowledge or demonstrates skills. The teacher thus instructs students in what to do and how best to do it.

Practical learning—The teacher demonstrates the steps or processes of undertaking specific tasks. Students observe the demonstration, discuss processes and skills used by the teacher and then practise these skills and processes in a familiar setting.

Experiential learning—The teacher plans for learning to take place in the field or place of work. Here students gain new knowledge as they practise skills in real-life situations. This teaching approach stresses the active participation of students in meaningful activities.

Teachers need to use a range of teaching methods to ensure students not only gain the process skills but can also apply them to relevant real-life situations. Teaching methods to develop these process skills include:

Brainstorming—These are activities that are planned to stimulate discussion amongst students, sharing ideas and opinions on how best to investigate, how best to tackle specific activities and so on.

Surveys and questionnaires—These investigative activities generally go hand in hand with brainstorming. Students collect, collate and analyse data so that they can make informed decisions. A questionnaire is a specific written form where people can record written responses to surveys.

Demonstrations—These integrate sources of information to show specific steps in completing tasks. The teacher demonstrates a process and identifies what research and reporting skills (including the source of information) were used to complete the task.

Discussion/seminars—These teaching methods allow students to clarify thoughts and present information in a logical order within a formal format (seminar) or a less formal format (group discussion). Through exposure to these processes, students develop a deeper understanding of issues/problems and can present informed possible solutions.

Problem-solving—This is a specific process that students can apply to investigate a task for which there is no immediate or obvious solution and establish an action plan to come up with a possible solution. The major steps in problem-solving tasks are:

1 identifying the problem
2 selecting or developing a strategy to solve the problem
3 implementing the devised plan
4 monitoring and recording results
5 evaluating the results

Presentations/reports—There are a variety of ways a teacher can organise presentations and reports. Reports may be part of a problem-solving task where students present their findings; this may be in oral or written form. They may be individual reports based on outcomes of specific investigative work (written or oral). Presentations by outside sources may be organised to present relevant information for students to use so that tasks can be completed, in particular large tasks such as projects.

Cooperative group work—The creation of democracy requires that people learn to work in groups Through carefully monitored group work, students can experience working as a team. Teachers need to:

- organise their classroom layout in such a way that cooperative learning is encouraged
- plan activities that require workers to work in pairs and small groups as well as individually
- construct activities where learners consult each other, share ideas and learn from each other. The content to be shared should not be predetermined by the teacher.

Project work—This allows the teacher to create real-life situations where students develop their understanding and skills. They also develop communication skills as they need to talk to each other to reach an understanding. As a group students have to use and apply basic research skills to locate relevant information as well as organised reporting skills to relay project outcomes. When devising projects teachers need to ensure that projects:

- use real-life or concrete examples
- encourage hands-on learning experiences
- are local and community based
- purposeful and meaningful learning experiences
- promote critical thinking and problem-solving
- encourage interaction with a range of individuals and contexts
- encourage active community participation

Planning

Planning, programming, assessing and reporting involve the consideration of the individual learning needs of all students and the creation of a learning environment that assists students to achieve the outcomes of the syllabus. Students' achievement of the syllabus outcomes is the goal of planning, programming and assessing. The sequence of learning experiences that teachers provide should build on what students already know and should be designed to ensure that they progress through the levels identified in the syllabus.

In an outcomes-based curriculum, lessons should be planned so that outcomes, assessment and classroom practice are all integrated. Assessment should not be tagged on to the end of a section of work but should be planned at the same time as planning the lesson content and should be ongoing.

Teaching programs need to be developed by teachers to structure learning experiences over a period of time. These programs should consist of:

A long-term plan—such as a yearly plan—where teachers identify and develop units of work that will be implemented over a long period of time. Teachers decide on the duration of these units of work in their long-term plan.

Short-term plans—These require the teacher to develop the units of work identified in the long-term plan. These units of work are generally planned to take 2–4 weeks.

Lesson plans—These are generally a further breakdown of the short-term plan (that is, the type of lessons that will be undertaken to achieve the short-term plan's objectives).

Planning guidelines

Plan groups of lessons that enable students to achieve the outcomes described in the syllabus. Fit each set of lessons into a short-term work plan. Use the table below as a checklist when planning lessons. Planning this way helps to align assessment with outcomes and with practicable teaching approaches in the classroom.

When planning, ask the focus questions:

- What do students need to know and what should they be able to do?
- What do they already know and what can they already do?
- How will I facilitate learning?
- How will I assess learning?

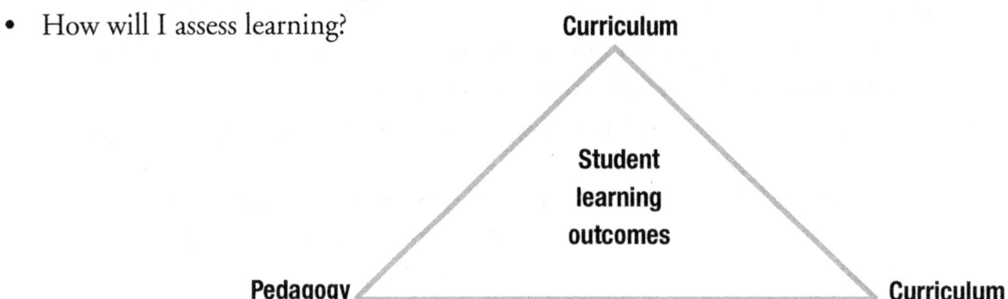

Lesson Planning Table

Outcomes	Things to plan for
1. Learning outcome or outcomes	Identify the outcome in the curriculum that you are working from.
2. Content: topic or key concept	To what theme do the lessons belong (e.g., Growing up)?
3. What will students learn in the particular lessons?	How will students achieve the learning outcome? List the appropriate • Knowledge to acquire • Skills to achieve • Values and attitudes to adopt
4. Number of lessons that need to be taught	How many lessons do you plan to teach on this particular topic?
Assessing progress	**Things to think through**
1. Evidence of learning	What you will look for in each learner's work? Write down the knowledge and skills that are to be assessed (each one should be something a learner can do).
2. The way learning will be assessed	Examples of what methods you may use: • formal (oral or written presentation • informal (teacher observation) • small task within a larger project • homework • test
Classroom practice	**Things to consider**
1. Method or activity	What will you and what will students do and in what sequence?
2. Time	For how long will you explain or demonstrate new concepts? For how long will students do each activity?
3. Teaching methods	How exactly will you arrange students? • as a whole group • working in pairs • working individually Where will students be? • in the classroom • outside
4. Resources needed	List any resources you may need for students to complete tasks

Assessment

Assessment should be an integral part of the teaching and learning process. Most teaching involves assessment, and by planning what to assess and recording the specific assessment information, appropriate assessment data can be collected.

There are a number of purposes for assessment.

- to collect and analyse information about students' learning
- to provide guidance, feedback and information about students' achievements and progress to both students and parents
- to inform program decision making and classroom organisational techniques

The most important purpose of assessment is to improve student learning. Assessment stems naturally from the teaching/learning situation. The assessment plan should be based on the outcomes from the syllabus. Teachers in their interaction with children constantly assess:

- students' current understandings
- the nature of any misconceptions
- students' current needs

Assessing and teaching cannot be separated, and assessment should inform teaching. Assessment is about finding out what students know and can do. The teacher constantly needs to ask:

- What do I want to know?
- How will I find out?

This should be an ongoing process as:

- assessing students continuously enables teachers to closely monitor and understand their progress.
- ongoing formal continuous assessment helps teachers diagnose problem areas in both learning and teaching, and allows teachers to adjust their teaching accordingly
- students receive helpful feedback after every assessment

Process of assessment

1 Provide students with opportunities to demonstrate what they know and can do in terms of identified learning outcomes.
2 Gather and record evidence of students' demonstration of learning outcomes.
3 Make judgments about students' demonstration of learning outcomes.

Assessment methods

The purpose, principles and processes of assessment are clearly described in the *Personal Development Teachers Guide* on pages 12–19. Assessment methods selected by the teacher should be appropriate to the situation and to the purpose of the assessment. Teachers have the opportunity to observe and record aspects of students' learning in a range of situations.

Group work—The teacher can determine the extent of student interaction and participation.

Listening—Listening to students respond to questions as well as other input, the teacher can collect many clues about students' current understanding and attitudes.

Interviewing students—Teachers can collect specific information about the way in which students think about certain situations. Other assessment methods can include:

- ➢ observation
- ➢ consultation
- ➢ analysis of students' work (examination of detailed evidence in student responses)
- ➢ self and peer assessment

Other sources of information for assessment purposes include the following:

- samples of students' work
- oral explanations or demonstrations to others
- questions posed by students
- practical tasks
- investigations and/or projects
- students' oral and written reports
- short quizzes
- pen and paper test

Reporting

Reporting is a way of communicating accurate information about students' demonstration of learning outcomes in a timely way. The purpose is to:

- acknowledge and support students' learning
- inform parents about the students' learning progress

Reporting modes include:

- written reports
- student teacher conferences
- parent interviews
- culminating performance or presentation
- portfolios

STRAND 1 Relationships

About this strand

We all belong to many different groups, and this strand is about the way we form relationships within those groups, such as our family, village, clan and church group. We all form different types of relationships within those groups and are expected to behave in certain ways. We have a number of reasons for forming different relationships and the worth or value in forming each one will vary. We also have rights as individuals within those relationships. Each person has a unique cultural and personal identity that is affected by the place they are from and the way they are brought up, so there are differences and similarities between people. As we get older we take on different roles and responsibilities and this affects our relationships, attitudes and behaviour. We all need to learn to manage and maintain our relationships, and this means that we need to share and be cooperative, to listen and be patient, tolerant and reasonable.

Sub-strands 1–4

Main ideas

Sub-strand 1: We all belong to different groups and within our relationships in those groups we behave in different ways.

Sub-strand 2: We all have a cultural and personal identity that depends on our origins and the influences on us.

Sub-strand 3: Our roles and responsibilities within our families change as we get older.

Sub-strand 4: Managing relationships requires skills such as sharing, being cooperative, listening, being positive, kind and patient.

Key words

Interactions, relationships, cultural identity, personal identity, communication skills, negotiation, conflict resolution, decision-making, self-esteem, roles, responsibilities, expectations, gender, culture, sexuality, adolescence, harassment, bullying

Assessment tasks

Assessment aims to gather information on how well students have achieved the outcomes of the Relationships strand. A variety of strategies should be used: written, oral and practical.

Each assessment item should be based on criteria that have been clearly written down. Students should be told what the criteria are so that they know the basis for judgment of their achievement and demonstration of the outcomes. In this way teachers will be able to measure how well the students have achieved the learning outcomes. Teachers should focus on the performance of each individual and be much less interested in comparing the performance of one student against another.

Assessment should also be continuous and collected throughout the learning process by the completion of appropriate activities such as those indicated with the assessment icon in the 'For you to try' sections.

Major links to other subjects

The Relationships strand builds upon ideas introduced in Culture and Community at the lower primary level. At the upper primary level, Relationships links to the substrand 'social and economic organisation' of Social Science and the substrand 'community development' of Making a Living. Aspects of different subjects can be integrated into activities such as:

- a project to improve relationships in the community
- collecting and analysing statistical data for specific groups in the community
- designing posters or performing a drama to relay the message of the benefits of positive relationships

Links with other subjects are noted with an icon in the student books.

Teacher information

Interactions in relationships and groups

A relationship is the way in which two or more people or groups behave towards each other and feel towards each other. The relationships that we have with other people are fundamental to the way we live in our families and in the community.

The groups to which we belong have an influence on the way we do things, dress and behave and on the ownership of property. In some societies property or other privileges may be passed on through the male line or through the female line, and may not be available to certain people. The way in which girls and women are valued also affects relationships. For example, in some cultures, women may be included in some decision-making processes but excluded from others.

We all belong to a family and there are different types of families. Most people in Papua New Guinea are living in villages in an extended family, although in more urban places the nuclear family is becoming more common. In some countries blended families are becoming more common, especially where people remarry after one partner dies or after a divorce and they bring the children from their respective marriages to live together in one household.

There are advantages and disadvantages to living in different kinds of family. For example:

Type of family	Advantages	Disadvantages
Extended family	Many people to help grow food, work, take care of children, take care of old people Language, culture and traditions are easily passed on If a child or other family member dies, there will still be many others in the family Children learn to respect culture and traditions	Many mouths to feed Many children to clothe and school fees to pay Women who have many children can get sick and die Children in large families may not be so healthy, especially when children are spaced close together
Nuclear family	Higher standard of living, easier to provide shelter, food, clothing, education Parents have more time and energy for their children	Children may not learn their culture and may not get to know some of their relatives Children may grow up to be selfish and not think about others Children may not learn to respect culture and traditions
Blended family	Parents have the opportunity to make a happy relationship with a new partner; for example, after the death of a partner or divorce. Children have the opportunity to be brought up by two parents. Children can learn patience, tolerance and understanding.	Children from different families may have conflict or rivalry with each other. Children may conflict with their stepmother or stepfather. Parents have two sets of children to provide and care for. A parent may conflict with children or stepchildren.
Polygamous family (e.g. polygyny)	A man has more than one wife to produce more children. A man has more than one wife to make gardens, raise pigs and other livestock, and farm cash crops. A man may have greater wealth and status because of his number of wives.	A man may need to provide a separate house for each wife. There may be conflict between the wives. A man may find it difficult to provide for all his wives and children.

Family members often take on or are given different roles and responsibilities. These roles and responsibilities are an important part of family interaction. Some examples are shown below:

Grandparents: help their children; teach and take care of grandchildren; pass on their knowledge, skills and experience to others; pass on traditional stories and beliefs and provide a link with previous generations.

Parents: teach and take care of their children; provide food, clothing and a loving and caring environment; set a good example for their children.

Sisters: play with and take care of younger sisters and brothers; learn from and respect older sisters and brothers.

Brothers: play with and take care of younger brothers and sisters; learn from and respect older brothers and sisters.

Aunts: take an active part in the family; act as role models for nieces and other girls and young women in the family; may play a special role in bringing up girls.

Uncles: take an active part in the family; act as role models for nephews and other boys and young men in the family; may play a special role in bringing up boys.

Cousins: are often friends and playmates for each other when they are children; give support and advice as they get older.

Relationship skills

When managing relationships, particular skills are needed in order for them to be effective and successful. For example:

Ways to maintain a healthy relationship	Skills needed
Gather information that is needed	Observing and asking questions Listening carefully Checking the accuracy and validity of information
Communicate well with each other	Listening Expressing yourself clearly Checking back with others to make sure that you understand them and that they understand you
Give and receive compliments (positive comments about each other)	Actively finding positive things to say about someone else to give recognition and acknowledgement Finding a suitable time and place to give the compliment Sincerity in your actions Allowing others to pay you a sincere compliment graciously and without either strongly denying or becoming too self-important as a result
Solve problems	Identifying the issue Thinking about alternative solutions Weighing up alternatives and choosing the best Evaluating the outcome
Weigh up information, make a decision and carry out the decision	Identifying criteria to evaluate different types of information
Other?	

Equality

In relationships between friends, and in other types of relationship, there should be equality. This means that both people in a relationship should be equally important and have the same amount of power. For example:

Examples of equality	Examples of inequality
Both people feel that they have the same amount of power, and share in giving their ideas	One person does most of the talking and the other person cannot give their point of view
Both people share in making decisions but can also accept the ideas of the other person	One person makes most of the important decisions while the other person is excluded or not involved
If shared money is involved, both have some influence and control over the way that money is spent	One person spends money belonging to both without consulting or knowing if the other person will agree
Both people have the capacity to be appropriately assertive	One person is overly assertive or aggressive and the other person is submissive
Both people treat the other person with dignity and respect, both in private and in public	One person makes the other look silly or is overly critical, both in private and in public
Both people are fairly independent and can cope with normal activities and decisions on their own	One person is heavily dependent on the other and cannot manage normal activities and decisions on his or her own.

Stereotyping and discrimination

Stereotyping occurs when we have a fixed general idea or image of a person and we expect the person to behave in that way, rather than waiting until we meet the person and then making up our own mind.

When we make up our minds without good reason and treat people unfairly then we are discriminating against that person. *Discrimination* is unfair and is against the law in many countries, including Papua New Guinea. For example, in some countries there is discrimination against people because of the colour of their skin, even though this is against the law.

Example of stereotyping or discrimination (Who was involved? What happened?)	**Why this is wrong and possible effect on the person**
Believing that a man is going to be aggressive because he is from the Highlands	We should not assume that all people from one place have the same characteristics. The man may feel he is being pre-judged and does not have the opportunity to show others what he is like.
Believing that a person will be lazy because she is from the coast	We should not assume that all people from one place have similar characteristics. The woman may feel that this is unfair and that she should not be included with other people from her province.
Thinking that someone from a remote or isolated area is not intelligent and does not understand complicated things	A person's intelligence is not decided by the place he comes from. The person may feel that others are laughing at him, which may hurt his self-esteem.
Thinking that someone is dishonest and not trustworthy because his clothes are dirty or untidy	The appearance of a person is not necessarily a good indication of his honesty.
Thinking that someone is honest and trustworthy because she is wearing smart clothes	A person who is well-dressed can sometimes be dishonest and try to trick others.
Thinking that someone is lazy because he or she is overweight	There may be other reasons why a person is overweight; for example, the person may not have a balanced diet or there may be genetic reasons.

Cultural and personal identity

The term 'culture' describes the way that people live in a particular place at a given time, and many of the ways that we use to describe ourselves come from our culture. Culture includes such things as our language, customs, ceremonies, beliefs and traditions; our stories, art, music and dance; the food that we grow and eat; the way we communicate; and the transport that we use.

In Papua New Guinea there are many different cultures although most of them share certain common characteristics. Many cultures in PNG maintain their traditions and appear to have changed little; however, all cultures change over time. For example, for traditional dancing, modern paints and other modern materials may be used together with feathers and leaves, or a temporary tattoo may be drawn with a marker pen rather than doing a permanent tattoo with a sharp thorn needle and tattoo paint. The coming of missionaries, traders, government and independence to PNG also had an impact on traditional cultures.

Traditionally, people in PNG live in groups whose sense of identity and loyalty does not extend beyond the village or language group that makes up the community. Important occasions in the life of the individual that are celebrated by the community include birth, initiation, marriage and death. The identity of men and women is usually determined by the special roles they have in their culture. Traditionally, men are warriors, hunters and protectors, and also do the heavy work of preparing new gardens. Women work in the gardens producing and cooking most of the food, and looking after children. These roles, however, are changing in modern society.

Membership of a clan also helps to give a sense of identity. Members of a clan are all descended from the same ancestor and usually remain loyal and helpful to one another even though they may live some distance apart. These extended families work together and share what they have as part of the wantok system.

In most cultures in PNG, people belong to their father's clan. These are known as patrilineal societies in which land and other property is passed on through the men. However, in some cultures in PNG, people belong to their mother's clan. These are matrilineal societies in which land and other possessions are passed on through the women of the clan. Examples of matrilineal societies are found in parts of the North Solomons and in the Trobriand Islands of Milne Bay.

Many clans have a special animal, bird or plant as their symbol or totem. People with the same totem may not be allowed to marry each other, although getting married and having children is usually important to the sense of identity of most men and women. Many men and women do not feel that they have achieved their full potential or purpose in life until they have had children. This feeling is further accentuated by societies that look on single or childless people as being somehow selfish or deserving of pity because they have no-one to whom they can pass their knowledge and skills and no-one to care for them in their old age and remember them when they have died.

In other societies, and increasingly in PNG, people are acquiring a sense of personal identity from their achievements at education and employment, and through the service and contribution that they provide to the community. For example, any work, including voluntary work, that we do in the community over a period of time that helps to make the community a better place should be acknowledged and remembered by the community and should also contribute to our sense of self-worth and identity.

Choosing positive role models

A role model is a person who is admired because of his or her personal qualities and the things that he or she has achieved. Role models are sometimes sporting heroes or musicians who are well known to the general public, but role models can also be people who quietly get on with their everyday lives. For example:

- people who have had many problems or unhappiness in their lives but continue to work cheerfully
- people who do voluntary work and who prefer to think about and help other people than to think so much about themselves
- people who come from a disadvantaged background but manage to overcome those disadvantages and achieve their goals
- people who are very good at what they do, but are still humble and modest and do not seek recognition or praise
- people who work very hard and achieve many things

Well-known sporting personalities are often seen as role models. Some possible reasons for choosing sportspeople as role models are listed in the examples of Dika Toua, the weightlifter, and Ryan Pini, the swimmer. People may have different reasons for choosing male and female role models.

Dika Toua:

- is the first woman from PNG to compete in weightlifting at the Olympic Games
- ranked sixth in the world at the Athens Olympic Games in 2004
- is very small—she is known as a 'pocket dynamo'
- is committed and dedicated; trains very hard every day ('eats, sleeps and breathes weightlifting')
- is following a dream
- has a special charm or appeal
- has very strong affection for her family and country—she is proud to represent PNG.

Ryan Pini:

- is very successful in his sport: he is one of the best in the Pacific; ranked eighteenth in the 100 m butterfly event at the Athens Olympics in 2004
- is self-confident
- tries hard to achieve his goals
- is disciplined and committed
- is friendly and easygoing
- gets on very well with other people.

Managing relationships—conflict resolution

Conflict in relationships is not unusual and may be inevitable. It helps to be prepared for conflict and have ways to deal with it when it arises. A group called the Conflict Resolution Network has developed a set of twelve tools to help people resolve conflict in their lives. These are briefly described in the box below.

The Twelve Tools of Conflict Resolution

1 **Win/win approach.** Conflict is seen as basically about differences in needs, attitudes and priorities. A win/win approach focuses on each person feeling that his or her needs, attitudes and priorities have been recognised and met to an acceptable level. This is unlike the win/lose or lose/lose interaction where one or both people are the losers, which is a disadvantage to group decision-making and the group itself.

2 **Creative response.** Creative response is about turning problems into challenges. Will you *react* or *respond*? It is best to choose to respond, to take charge and steer. Acknowledge the situation for what it is. Accept that you cannot be right all the time and that others cannot be perfect, but don't let go of your desire for change.

3 **Empathy—opening up or closing down communication.** Empathy involves recognising the motivation and feelings behind the attitudes and behaviour of others or putting yourself in their shoes.

4 **Appropriate assertiveness.** This involves expressing your needs, attitudes and priorities clearly, in neutral terms and not being defensive. Good conflict resolution requires you to be able to state your case without arousing the defences of the other person. We need to recognise the differences between aggressive, passive and assertive behaviour.

5 **Cooperative power.** Cooperative power requires focusing on the difference between power *over* someone else and power *with* someone else.

6 **Managing emotions.** This includes handling personal anger, frustration, sadness and grief.

7 **Willingness to resolve.** Willingness to resolve the issue relies on an understanding of how resentment makes good working relationships more difficult.

8 **Mapping the conflict.** Mapping the conflict involves being clear about the underlying needs, values, priorities and objectives of all those involved. Writing these down provides a 'map' of similarities, differences and which issues to focus on.

9 **Designing options.** Design answers that create wins for everyone.

10 **Negotiation skills.** This involves trying to create a problem-solving environment and working together towards resolution, ensuring therefore that the problem or issue is the 'enemy' and not the people involved.

11 **Third party mediations.** This involves using a third party as mediator for both 'sides'.

12 **Broadening perspectives.** Developing a broader perspective on the issue requires a recognition that others have a valid point of view.

STRAND 2

Movement and Physical Activity

About this strand

This strand introduces the movement skills needed in a range of physical activities, games, dance and sport. Students learn to link a range of locomotor and non-locomotor skills in sequences and to use and adapt this range of skills to form tactics and strategies. Learning and using these movement skills will help in the development of physical fitness which is good for health. There are risks involved in any physical activity and these can be reduced by following the rules and safety procedures, and also by developing ways to deal with unsafe or emergency situations.

Everyone can benefit from leisure and recreation activities but strategies are needed to encourage participation and to increase or improve the availability of resources. People must take on different roles and responsibilities in games and sports in order for them to run well. During team games, the players and officials must communicate and cooperate.

Sub-strands 1–5

Main ideas

Sub-strand 1: Movement skills include locomotor skills and non-locomotor skills that are combined in sequences and form part of strategies when we play sport.

Sub-strand 2: Physical activities help to promote physical fitness, which is good for health.

Sub-strand 3: Rules and safety procedures help to prevent injury when people are playing sport.

Sub-strand 4: Leisure and recreation are important for our health and well-being, but the options available depend on the facilities and opportunities in each area.

Sub-strand 5: In order for sports and games to run effectively people must take on different roles and responsibilities, and these will affect our attitudes, relationships and behaviour.

Key words

Movement skill, movement patterns, locomotor, non-locomotor, coordination, tactics, strategies, fitness, health, performance, body shape, leisure, recreation, relationships, roles, responsibilities, planning, coordinating, implementing, promoting

Assessment tasks

Assessment aims to gather information on how well students have achieved the outcomes of the Movement and Physical Activity strand. A variety of strategies should be used: practical, written and oral. For this strand there should also be direct observation of the development of the ten skills in the seven modified sports.

Each assessment item should be based on criteria that have been clearly written down. Students should be told what the criteria are so that they know the basis for judgment of their achievement and demonstration of the outcomes. In this way teachers will be able to measure how well the students have achieved the learning outcomes. Teachers should focus on the performance of each individual and be much less interested in comparing the performance of one student against another.

Assessment should also be continuous and collected throughout the learning process by the completion of appropriate activities such as those indicated with the assessment icon in the 'For you to try' sections.

For more information about assessment of Movement and Physical Activity, refer to the Modified Sports manual.

Major links to other subjects

The Movement and Physical Activity strand builds upon ideas introduced in Health and Physical Education at the lower primary level. At the upper primary level, Movement and Physical Activity links to the substrand 'people and environment' of Social Science, the substrand 'skills development' of Arts and the substrand 'better living' of Making a Living. Aspects of different subjects can be integrated into activities such as:

- a project to improve sporting facilities and opportunities in the community
- collecting and analysing statistical data for specific sporting groups or teams in the community
- designing posters or performing a drama to relay the message of the benefits of sport

Links with other subjects are noted as an icon in the student books.

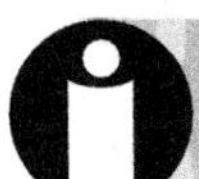

Teacher information

In all games and sports, the importance of movement skills, fitness and safety should be emphasised consistently throughout, so that students can improve their skills, improve or maintain their health and minimise the risk of injury.

At primary level, modified sports become the focus of the Movement and Physical Activity strand. At lower primary, students play various sports using modified rules, skills, fields, number of players etc. At upper primary, they begin to learn the adult version of the sporting codes. There should be a gradual move from modified sports to adult sport with appropriate skills, rules, tactics and so on. The movement skills (locomotor and non-locomotor), sequences, patterns, knowledge of safety procedures, and so on, all need to be acquired in order to be able to play sports and games at the higher level.

Fitness for health

Health can be encouraged through a range of fitness activities. Students should be encouraged to take part both in competitive sports and a range of non-competitive or cooperative activities to improve health and fitness. Some examples are listed below.

Non-competitive activities

- ➢ Sweeping leaves
- ➢ Working in the garden
- ➢ Emptying rubbish bins
- ➢ Walking
- ➢ Cutting grass
- ➢ Collecting rubbish and cleaning up
- ➢ Swimming
- ➢ Planting fruit trees

Modified sports

In Papua New Guinea there are seven modified sports that have been adapted especially for young people and a number of basic skills that are used in each sport.

Modified sports

Modified sport	Basic skills
Kapul soka (soccer)	• dribbling, stopping • trapping • passing or kicking, striking • heading, goalkeeping • tackling • throwing in
Tibol (softball)	• throwing • catching • fielding • pitchin • batting • base running
Mini-basketball	• passing • catching • dribbling • shooting • bouncing and re-bouncing
Netabol (netball)	Ball handling skills • one-handed shoulder pass • two-handed chest pass • lob throw • bounce pass, side pass • shooting • catching Attacking skills • catching on the run • catching and pivoting • throwing and dodging (*cont.*)
Netabol (netball) (*cont.*)	Defending skills • shadowing • intercepting the ball • blocking • defending a shot or pass
Pukpuk ragbi (rugby)	• passing • tagging • running with the ball • sidestepping • running forward, evading and spinning • dummy passing • chip kicking • fending
Mini-volleyball	• the serve • the dig • the set or volley • the spike • the block
Liklik cricket	Skills • batting • catching • bowling • wicketkeeping • fielding Tactics • batting • bowling • fielding

Helping other people

Competition in sport can be a useful way of motivating players to improve their skills but, when people become too concerned with winning, they sometimes behave unreasonably and may do silly things. Students should be encouraged to focus on improving their own performance, rather than being concerned with always winning or beating the opposition. They could think of ways they can measure improvements in their individual performance so that they are competing against themselves rather than other people. In this way, by measuring their improvement, all players can get a sense of achievement. This is what athletes and other sportspeople often refer to as their 'Personal Best' or 'PB'.

Sports injuries

Prevention

All physical activity involves some risk, but accidents and injuries can be prevented in the following ways:

- Keep yourself fit.
- Don't play if you are ill (for example, with malaria, diarrhoea or a cold).
- Don't play if you have an injury that has not completely healed, such as a sprained muscle.
- Cover any sores or cuts.
- Take it easy, or stop the activity if you get hurt or feel pain.
- Have lots of sleep and rest.
- Eat good food and drink plenty of water so that you do not become dehydrated, especially when playing sport during the daytime.
- When you have been ill or injured, return to the activity slowly and progressively.
- Warm up and stretch carefully before being very active.
- Choose activities that suit your level of skill and fitness.
- Wear suitable clothing for the activity.
- Keep all equipment in good condition.
- If necessary, support your ankles (for example, by using tape).
- If you are hurt, get advice quickly from a health worker.
- Know your limits—try your best, but don't go too far.
- Be positive in your thinking and behaviour.
- Avoid dangerous play and do not fool around.
- Never use alcohol or other drugs before or during physical activity.
- Cooperate with others in the team.
- Know and obey the rules of the game.
- Obey the referee's or umpire's decision even if you disagree.
- Make sure that all fixtures such as goalposts are secure and won't fall over.
- Check that the playing area is level with no holes or dips.
- Make sure that spectators are kept well back from the edge of the playing area and do not enter the area at any time.
- Warn spectators and other participants about balls or other flying objects (for example, discus) that can injure people.
- Learn some first aid.
- Keep water, ice (if available), clean cloths and a first aid kit close to the playing area.

Stretching

Stretching before any physical activity will greatly reduce the risk of injury. Slow, careful stretches of each set of muscles will help to lengthen the muscle in preparation for the activity. Stretching helps relax the muscle, improves blood circulation and improves performance. You should do the following:

- Warm up by walking or jogging before stretching.
- Stretch before and after the activity.
- Stretch each set of muscles to be used.
- Stretch gently and slowly.
- Never bounce or stretch rapidly.
- Stretch until you feel tension or discomfort but never pain.
- Breathe slowly and regularly throughout stretching—do not hold your breath.

Treatment

Soft tissue injuries

Soft tissue injuries include injuries to skin, muscles and some ligaments. These injuries can be treated by using the sequence of activities known as **RICE**:

- **R**—rest the injured part.
- **I**—wrap some ice in cloth to make an ice pack and place it firmly over the injured body part. If ice is not available very cold water can be used.
- **C**—wrap a firm compression bandage over, above and below the injury site.
- **E**—elevate the site so that it is higher than, or at the same level as, the heart.

Soft tissue injury (no broken skin)	**Treatment**
Bruise—bleeding inside the muscle	Use ice for twenty minutes and reapply every two hours for first twenty-four hours. Do not rub.
Sprain—the ligaments that hold a joint are torn. Painful, unable to move. Common in soccer, rugby, basketball, netball and softball.	Use RICE and bandage and splint the joint so that it cannot move. Get medical help.
Strain—an overstretched muscle or tendon	Use RICE.

Other soft tissue injuries	**Treatment**
Eye injuries—small loose objects in the eye (may be washed out naturally by tears)	Get the person to look up and carefully remove the object with the corner of a clean cloth, or gently wash the eye with a stream of clean water.
Cramps—occur when muscles are overused, jarred, lose body salt or have poor blood supply	Gently stretch the muscle. Apply an ice pack. Do not massage.
Stitch—cramping of the muscles of the ribcage or diaphragm when running	Slow down, breathe deeply, rest.
Winding—hard to breathe after being hit in the upper abdomen	Lay down in comfortable position. Do not pump the legs or rub where the person was hit.
Groin and testicle injuries	Lay back in a comfortable position. Apply an ice pack. Do not urinate.
External bleeding	Apply direct pressure. Place a clean dressing or cloth over the wound. Place a bigger cloth or pad over that and bandage firmly. Raise and rest the injured part.
Internal bleeding—coughing up frothy blood, or passing urine or faeces streaked with blood	Rest in a comfortable position. Loosen clothes. Don't let the person eat or drink. Get medical help.
Abrasions—tearing the skin by falling on the ground. If dirty, the wound may become infected.	Clean thoroughly with a very clean cloth soaked in clean water. Cover with a dressing or very clean cloth. If something is sticking out from a deep wound, control the bleeding by applying pressure to the surrounding area and get medical help urgently.

Note: When dealing with injuries that involve blood and open wounds, you should wash your hands before and after helping the person. As far as possible you should not touch blood or the wound. If you do get blood on your skin, then you should wash it off with plenty of water.

Hard tissue injuries

Hard tissue injuries involve bones and cartilage that can be hurt during sports and take a long time to heal.

Hard tissue injury	Treatment
Fractures—breakage of a bone, which may cause loss of blood. Very painful, with loss of power and movement.	Support the fractured part with bandages and/or splints. Broad bandages or cloths are best and should not be too tight or too loose. Splints can be thin branches, bamboo or a school ruler, but need to be a little longer than the bone. Use padding to stop the splint rubbing or cutting the body. Tie broad cloths around the limb and splint so that it cannot move. Get medical help.
Head injuries—which may include concussion or the person being unconscious.	Even if the person appears to be all right they should stop playing. Get medical advice. If the person is unconscious, place them on their side and check that the air passages are clear, that the person is breathing and that they have a pulse. Support the head and neck if you have to move the person. Get medical help urgently.

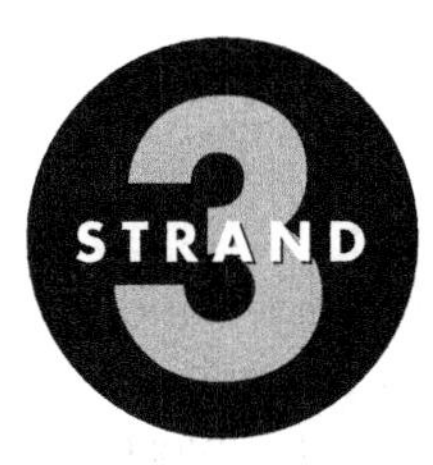

Our Culture, Lifestyle and Values

About this strand

This strand looks at the value of customs, rituals and traditions associated with different cultural groups and their influence on family and community life and contribution to national identity. Students will explore the effect on lifestyle of physical and economic changes in the environment and outline the elements of the lifestyle they would prefer in the future.

Sub-strands 1–2

Main ideas

Sub-strand 1: Culture and values, their influence on family and community life and contribution to national identity.

Sub-strand 2: Changes in the physical and economic environment and the effect on community lifestyle over time.

Key words

Culture, customs, celebrations, roles, responsibilities, lifestyle, values, beliefs, symbols, rituals, traditions, cultural practices, religious practices, respect, acceptance, opportunities, choices, physical environment, economic environment

Assessment tasks

Assessment aims to gather information on how well students have achieved the outcomes of the Our Culture, Lifestyle and Values strand. A variety of strategies should be used: written, oral and practical.

Each assessment item should be based on criteria that have been clearly written down. Students should be told what the criteria are so that they know the basis for judgment of their achievement and demonstration of the outcomes. In this way teachers will be able to measure how well the students have achieved the learning outcomes. Teachers should focus on the performance of each individual and be much less interested in comparing the performance of one student against another.

Assessment should also be continuous and collected throughout the learning process by the completion of appropriate activities such as those indicated with the assessment icon in the 'For you to try' sections.

Major links to other subjects

The Our Culture, Lifestyle and Values strand builds upon ideas introduced in Culture and Community at the lower primary level. At the upper primary level, Our Culture, Lifestyle and Values links to the substrands 'cultural expression' of Social Science, the substrand 'creativity and responding to the arts' of Arts and the substrand 'making things' of Making a Living. Aspects of different subjects can be integrated into activities such as:

- a project to involve a variety of people in one aspect of the life in the community
- collecting and analysing statistical data for specific groups or activities in the community
- designing posters or performing a drama to relay the message of the benefits of an aspect of community life

Links with other subjects are noted as an icon in the student books.

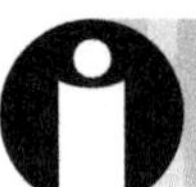

Teacher information

Traditions in a changing society

Traditions are still very strong in Papua New Guinea but changes are also taking place. One example is the way the people communicate. In the Highlands, people were often separated by deep valleys but called from hilltop to hilltop. In this way a message could be passed easily over a long distance. In some parts of the country, such as the Sepik, the garamut or slit drum was used to send a message to people outside the village. Many coastal people make a hole in a conch shell, which they then blew, in order to send a message. In many communities these methods of communication are still used but more modern methods have also been introduced. For example, the postal service sends letters and parcels from one part of the country to another and also overseas. Radio and telephone are also an important method of communication in PNG. More recently, computers with email and mobile phones mean that people in some parts of the country are able to communicate immediately with people all over the world.

Bride price in a changing society

Bride price involves the exchange of goods between clans of a man and a woman as they get married. Bride price is important to the community because it helps to develop, improve and maintain the relationship between clans of the man and the woman who are marrying each other. In many parts of PNG the man's clan usually gives goods and money to the bride's clan. In other areas—for example, the Trobriand Islands of Milne Bay—the bride gives goods to the man's clan and, in return, the bride's clan receives money for the goods paid. Bride price has been an important part of PNG culture for many generations and should not be seen as a way to obtain wealth. The payment of bride price achieves the following purposes:

- it recognises a relationship between a man and woman
- it is an agreement, promise and contract between two clans of a couple (husband and wife)
- it is a confirmation of marriage between two clans.

The bride price is usually paid in a number of different forms. As well as traditional items such as pigs and other animals, food, pottery, betel nuts and shell money, bride price today can include thousands of kina and trade store goods. Some people feel that the size of bride price payments in some places has become too large and that it is more like a competition between clans or villages than an important tradition that helps to hold people together in a significant relationship. Some people may feel that bride price has no relevance in a modern society, but all societies change with time and communities can still maintain the significance of bride price if they choose to do so.

Funerals

Funeral ceremonies are important occasions in Papua New Guinea. For example, in New Ireland Province malanggan is one of the death ceremonies still being celebrated, although malanggan also describes the sacred objects that go with the ceremony. The purpose of the ceremony is to remember the person who has died and to mark the initiation into the clan of an adolescent boy who will replace the one who has died. The ceremony may take many years to prepare, needing extra gardens to be planted and pigs to be bought or raised. The carvings and other objects show people, flowers, fish and crocodiles and mythical creatures in great detail and are brightly painted. Some are carved from tree trunks, like totem poles. Other objects are made from cane, like baskets, and are covered in shells and feathers. The malanggan ceremony unites the people as they do all the hard work and preparation that is needed. During the time leading up to the ceremony, people still feel sad but slowly begin to accept that the person has died.

Amongst the Binandere people of the Oro Province, the widow or widower goes away from the group and makes a special jacket and other body ornaments from the seeds known as Job's tears and these are worn at the funeral ceremony. During this time the men go hunting and fishing and the meat and fish are smoked so that they can be kept for a big feast. During the ceremony to honour the dead person a special dance and drama called an ario is performed.

Although the dances, music and traditions of each culture differ, the reasons behind death ceremonies are similar. People express their grief and sorrow at the death of their loved one in a traditional way, and this a healthy thing to do and helps people to accept the death. In some places people rub mud on their bodies and sing songs of mourning. If people think that the death was caused by sorcery, then these songs may express hostility towards their enemies.

Although Papua New Guinea is changing, funeral ceremonies still have an important part to play in the way of life of the community. If someone dies outside their own province, the family will often go to much trouble and expense to carry the body home so that the funeral can be conducted according to the wishes of the family.

The environment in a changing society

Living things and our surroundings provide the basis for our way of life and culture. Our resources include mountains, rivers, lagoons, plants, animals and agricultural systems. If we do not look after these resources and our surroundings, we will lose part of our culture that we value so much. We need air, water, soil, plants and animals. For these reasons, we need to have an understanding of ecology (the study of how living things interact with each other and with their non-living surroundings).

Our traditional understanding of the environment helps us to continue to provide food and shelter and be able to reproduce. Agriculture and the collection of other foods depend on understanding and respecting the ecology of the country. Land and sea resources must be used carefully if we want a productive world for people in the future.

We have a responsibility to leave a living, productive world for others to enjoy. Papua New Guineans understand the spiritual importance of plants, animals and other natural resources. In many places these are protected in a number of ways. It is right and proper to continue to respect living things and their surroundings. It is wrong and foolish to think that these resources are there only for people to use and destroy. Our ideas of beauty are also based on what we see in living things and the surroundings. If we destroy or spoil these things then the result is an ugly world.

There are many types of plants and animals in Papua New Guinea that are found nowhere else in the world. Many of these plants and animals have not been studied properly to understand their special place in the ecology of our environment. Once these plants and animals are studied, our understanding of them will increase and they may prove to be useful as medicines or in other ways. For example, quinine, which is a medicine for malaria, comes from the bark of the cinchona tree that grows in tropical rainforests. Throughout the world, rainforests are being rapidly destroyed, threatening traditional cultures and reducing the range of living things. In Papua New Guinea, forests are threatened by population growth, the growth of the cash economy, and poor logging practices.

We cannot leave living things and their surroundings to take care of themselves because of the very rapid increase in the human population and the effects of modern technology. Humans are the most powerful force on the earth and have the ability to affect the plants and animals, the rivers and the seas. As we try to improve the quality of our lives, we are changing and sometimes destroying the systems of agriculture, the ways of using resources and traditional knowledge. These ways have guided us and supplied our needs for thousands of years. We need to understand that we can work with the environment to improve it, or we will damage it due to our short-sighted behaviour.

Lifestyles in a changing environment

Thousands of years ago, human beings were able to supply their needs for food, clothing and shelter from their surroundings. They hunted wild animals and gathered useful plants. They also used non-living things such as rocks, fire and water. At this time, the human population was small and because of the way people lived they did not have a serious effect on other living things or on the surroundings. A few traditional societies still live in this way today.

About 10 000 years ago, in Papua New Guinea and in other parts of the world, an important change took place. Agriculture began and people were no longer just hunters and gatherers. The beginning of agriculture meant that people began to have a greater impact on the environment. One of the earliest agricultural sites in the world has been found in the Kuk swamp in the Wahgi valley of the Western Highlands Province. In 1998, the Kuk archaeological site was nominated for recognition as a World Heritage Site.

Today, people are able to live a different way of life because they have developed agriculture, mining and industry to meet the needs of a large population. This development means that more living things are consumed and more non-living things are taken from the surroundings. The activities of modern societies also produce wastes that can damage living things and pollute the environment. Due to the rapid growth in population, the activities of humans are having an increasingly large impact on the environment. Many of these effects can destroy living things and their surroundings, which together are known as **ecosystems.**

All societies affect their environment by farming the land, harvesting the forest, fishing the seas and mining the earth. People do this to provide for the many essential needs relating to survival and to improve the quality of life. As the world population increases, these needs will also increase. So that the environment continues to provide these resources and is not destroyed, people must look after it and manage it well.

By using sensible management policies and procedures that apply the principles of ecology, the stability of the environment can be maintained. The diversity of an environment is a very important factor in maintaining stability. When an environment contains a variety of living things, it is more likely to be stable.

Protected areas

In order to make responsible use of the environment and to care for it, certain areas of Papua New Guinea have been protected for different reasons, such as public use, education, conservation and research. Examples of protected areas are shown in the following table.

Protected area	Description
National parks	Large areas (greater than 2000 ha) for educational and recreational purposes, e.g. Varirata, at Sogeri outside Port Moresby. Eventually, it is planned to have a national park to represent every type of environment in the country.
Provincial parks	Small areas (less than 2000 ha) of scenic and recreational importance near urban areas, e.g. Mt Gahavisuka outside Goroka, Eastern Highlands.
Historical sites	Areas of historical importance, e.g. Cape Wom, outside Wewak, East Sepik Province.
Nature reserves	Representative areas set aside to protect wildlife, ecosystems and habitats, with some research and limited access, e.g. Talele Island, East New Britain Province.
National walking track	The Kokoda Track, Oro Province and Central Province.
Sanctuaries	Areas for research, wildlife breeding programs, and public viewing of wildlife, e.g. Baiyer River, Western Highlands Province.
Wildlife management areas	Areas set up at the request of landowners, who retain ownership, for conservation and sustainable use of wildlife and ecosystems, e.g. the Hunstein Range, East Sepik Province. (For more information on forest management in the Hunstein, see page 43 of the Papua New Guinea Secondary School Atlas.)
World Heritage Sites	Areas of environmental or cultural significance to the whole world. In 1998, the Kuk archaeological site in the Western Highlands was nominated for recognition as a World Heritage Site.

National animals

The animals that are found in Papua New Guinea and Australia are unique because they have evolved separately from the animals in South-East Asia. About 50 000 years ago, the sea level was lower than today and so Australia and Papua New Guinea were joined together. However, PNG was never joined to Asia, so the animals are different in Asia. One of the main differences is the presence of marsupials or mammals that have a pouch. For example, there are marsupials such as wallabies, cuscus and tree kangaroos in Papua New Guinea, but not in South-East Asia. The line that separates the animals of South-East Asia from the animals of Papua New Guinea and Australia runs through the islands of Indonesia close to the mainland and is called the **Wallace Line.**

Some animals in Papua New Guinea are thought to be so unique, in danger of extinction or in need of protection that they have been protected by law. These animals are called national animals. They cannot be used for commercial purposes, although some can be hunted by traditional methods for traditional purposes. National animals are listed in the following table.

National animals of PNG	Examples	
Birds of paradise	King bird of paradise Lawes' parotia Kissaba Superb bird of paradise Trumpet manucode Brown sickle-billed bird of paradise	Short-tailed paradigalla Magnificent bird of paradise Blue bird of paradise Emperor bird of paradise Red bird of paradise
Other birds	New Guinea eagle Goura pigeons Large egret Salvadori's teal Osprey	
Other animals	Long-snouted echidna Boelen's python Birdwing butterflies Dugong	

Suggested activities: Managing the environment

The following table shows the effect of mining on the Ok Tedi and Fly Rivers. A, B and C are three points on the river system, with point A being the furthest upstream and point C being the furthest downstream. Dead areas are places where the trees and other living things have been killed, unless they could move out of the area. Stressed areas are places where the trees and other plants are unhealthy or dying.

Damage caused by flooding from blocked rivers (in square kilometres)

Dead areas			
Year	**A (furthest upstream)**	**B**	**C (furthest downstream)**
1992	5.5	0.0	0.0
1995	16.8	0.3	0.2
1996	29.1	8.5	0.4
Stressed areas			
Year	**A (furthest upstream)**	**B**	**C (furthest downstream)**
1992	11.7	0.3	0.0
1995	24.8	7.6	3.0
1996	20.6	32.1	15.2

Sources: Papua New Guinea Primary School Atlas, p. 36 and Papua New Guinea Secondary School Atlas, p. 40, Oxford University Press

1. How would you describe the amount of damage in all three places (A, B and C) in 1992?
2. How would you describe the changes in dead areas in all three places (A, B and C) from 1992 to 1996?
3. How would you describe the changes in stressed areas in all three places (A, B and C) from 1992 to 1996?
4. Overall, how would you describe the trend or pattern of the changes in all three places (A, B and C) from 1992 to 1996?

Reasons for changes in lifestyle

Papua New Guinea changed with the arrival of the European missionaries, traders and government officials. Examples of changes that occurred are:

- The missionaries taught religion so the teachings of the elders were seen as less important.
- The traders had things to sell for which people needed money, so planting of cash crops became a way to earn money.
- In order to earn money, people sometimes left their area in order to work in plantations, the public service and private enterprise.

- The kiaps or patrol officers who worked for the government stopped tribal and other fighting. Warriors, traditional teachers and leaders then played a less important part in community life.

Settlement patterns

In Papua New Guinea about 85 per cent of the people live in rural areas but one of the recent changes that has taken place in the lifestyle of people is in the growth of towns.

The way that houses are arranged in a village or a town is called the **settlement pattern**. In rural areas where the land is poor and cannot support a large population, people often live in isolated settlements. Sometimes settlements are scattered and there is no distinct pattern. This is called a **dispersed settlement** or **scattered settlement**. Sometimes the settlement stretches along a transport route such as road, river or coastline in a **linear settlement**. Sometimes the settlement spreads outwards from a centre in a **radial settlement**. Another type of settlement is a **nuclear settlement** that develops around a road junction, cultural centre or some other natural resource. Businesses often start in a nuclear settlement, which provide goods and services to the community and also allow people to earn money.

Nuclear settlements can develop into towns or cities that then have their own settlement pattern. For example, Port Moresby is a city that has a number of separate centres for government, administration, business, industry and shopping. The residential areas are spread between these centres.

Advantages and disadvantages of urban life

Living in a town or city might seem attractive, but there are both positive and negative aspects of this choice.

Advantages	Disadvantages
greater variety of possible employment	no work may be available, or workers may need special skills
many things to see and do	no land to grow food or the land may have poor soil
greater variety of people	crime rates may be higher
provision of services such as electricity and piped water	people need money to buy food, goods and services
greater variety of food available	the town/city may be too crowded
greater variety of shops	noisy
different kinds of entertainment—television, sports, dancing	houses are expensive

The story 'Moale comes to town' in Student Book 2 illustrates a range of physical, economic and social changes taking place in different parts of her province as a result of a new oil palm plantation, logging and a small mine. Examples of these changes are shown in the table below.

Physical changes	Economic changes	Social changes
old coconut plantation cut down; oil palm planted	people paid money in royalties (but maybe not as much as they expect)	more traffic accidents
previously clean river now muddy	village people earning money selling fruit and vegetables	children caught stealing
large trees being cut down—changing the environment	men spending money on drinking	men drink more and women feel less safe
new roads built	greater choice of goods to buy	more jobs (but mainly for people with skills)
new market, hospital, department store, mine		hospital short of equipment and staff—has not improved health service

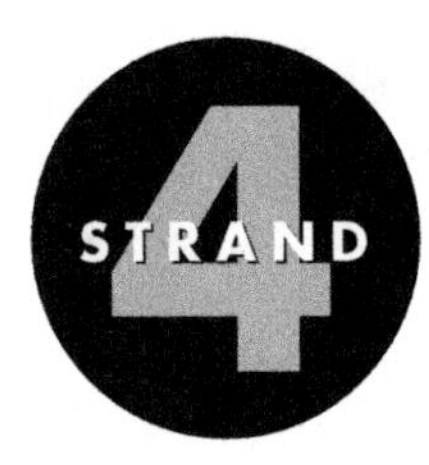

Health of Individuals and Populations

About this strand

The overall purpose of this strand is to introduce students to the knowledge, skills and attitudes they need in order to be a healthy individual and a member of a healthy community. Students will acquire knowledge about growth and development, nutrition, personal health and safety, community health and the use of drugs. Students will learn to analyse and evaluate information in order to become informed. They will learn the skills required to make informed choices about issues that affect their health and safety since it is often the choices that we make about the way that we live that affect our health. This approach to health can be summarised by the expression 'Prevention is better than cure'. The strand also encourages the development of appropriate attitudes and ethical values in relation to human sexuality.

Sub-strands 1–5

Main ideas

Sub-strand 1: The physical, social and emotional changes that take place during growth and development, and the influences on those changes.

Sub-strand 2: Nutrition and its application to the way that people plan and prepare meals to achieve a balanced diet.

Sub-strand 3: Factors affecting the personal health and safety of the community, including common illnesses and diseases and health problems caused by our behaviour.

Sub-strand 4: Community health issues and concerns such as environmental health and communicable diseases such as HIV/AIDS.

Sub-strand 5: The use of drugs, both as medicine and for recreation, and their beneficial and harmful effects.

Assessment tasks

Assessment aims to gather information on how well students have achieved the outcomes of the Health of Individuals and Populations strand. A variety of strategies should be used: written, oral and practical.

Each assessment item should be based on criteria that have been clearly written down. Students should be told what the criteria are so that they know the basis for judgment of their achievement

Key words

Growth, development, infancy, childhood, puberty, adolescence, sexuality

Nutrition, carbohydrates, fats, proteins, vitamins, fibre, food groups, balanced diet, food preparation, food handling, staple food

Health promotion, hygiene, signs and symptoms, risks, hazards, behaviour, HIV/AIDS, sexually transmitted infections, peer pressure, dignity, respect, ethical values

Drugs, medicines, prescription drugs, non-prescription drugs, betel nut, tobacco, alcohol, marijuana

and demonstration of the outcomes. In this way teachers will be able to measure how well the students have achieved the learning outcomes. Teachers should focus on the performance of each individual and be much less interested in comparing the performance of one student against another.

Assessment should also be continuous and collected throughout the learning process by the completion of appropriate activities such as those indicated with the assessment icon in the 'For you to try' sections.

Major links to other subjects

The Health of Individuals and Populations strand builds upon ideas introduced in Health at the lower primary level. At the upper primary level, Health of Individuals and Populations links to the substrand 'people and environment' and 'societies and communities' of Social Science, and the substrands 'healthy living' of Making a Living. Aspects of different subjects can be integrated into activities such as:

- a health project to care for our body
- collecting and analysing statistical data for specific diseases
- designing posters to relay the message of healthy living
- reading and planning recipes
- measuring ingredients for specific purposes
- designing healthy eating plans

Links with other subjects are noted as an icon in the student books.

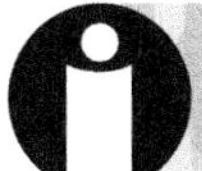

Teacher information

What is health?

There are a number of definitions of health, but the World Health Organization describes health as 'a state of complete physical, mental and social well-being and not merely the absence of disease or infirmity'. One of the main messages of health workers everywhere is that 'Prevention is better than cure'. This means that it is best to avoid a health problem if we can, rather than wait until we get sick and then look for treatment. However, when a person does get sick it is important for the person to seek treatment from a health worker quickly and not to wait until the problem gets worse.

Growth and development

The growth and development of a human being moves through a sequence of stages: infancy, childhood, puberty and adolescence into adulthood and old age. The progression from one stage to another is also known as the 'life cycle'.

Important ways to care for the body are eating a balanced diet, keeping our bodies and our surroundings clean, taking exercise, and not smoking, chewing betel nut with lime or drinking too much. More importantly, we should put these ideas into practice. It is particularly important to apply our knowledge to our behaviour in everyday life. There is little point in knowing how to care for the body if we do not do it every day since knowledge alone will not help us to be healthy.

Influences on our growth and development can be inherited or environmental. Inherited characteristics come from our genes, contained in the egg and sperm that came from our parents. This information decides characteristics such as our appearance and intelligence, although these are also influenced by environmental factors. Examples of environmental factors are physical living conditions, social and emotional factors (support from family and friends) and intellectual factors (the information we obtain).

Children usually inherit physical features from their parents, although there are often differences between children and parents too. Children may also have similar personality characteristics to their parents, although children can be quite different to their parents in personality. Examples of inherited physical features and personality characteristics are listed below.

Physical features

- shape of nose
- colour of skin
- type of hair
- height and weight
- body shape

Personality characteristics

- sense of humour
- easygoing nature
- talkative
- generous
- friendly
- strict
- quiet
- positive
- happy
- optimistic

Sexual development

Although it is natural and healthy to be interested in sex, sources of information about sexual development are not always easily available or reliable. This topic is sensitive and some teachers may find this difficult; yet the school may be the only place where young people get reliable information. Young people who have reliable information can protect themselves against unwanted pregnancy and sexually transmitted infections (STIs) by applying the information to their behaviour. Research in a number of countries has shown that people who have sex education do not go out and experiment with sex, but wait until later in their lives before they start to have sex. So this is a good reason for teachers to deal with this topic. Educating girls has also been shown to improve the health of children since educated girls usually delay the first pregnancy and have fewer and healthier children.

Different parts of the reproductive system have different functions in the process of conception or fertilisation. For example, the testicles hang outside the body in the scrotum where it is a little cooler and this helps the body to produce sperm. At the end of sexual intercourse, sperm are ejaculated in the vagina and must swim through the cervix into the uterus and then into the Fallopian tube (or oviduct) in order for fertilisation to occur. Fertilisation can only take place in the Fallopian tube and if there is no egg present then fertilisation cannot occur. This means that a woman can only conceive for a few days each month when she is fertile. For most women this is usually about fourteen days after the end of the last period. Some women notice that the vagina produces clear, slippery mucus at this time, and they can use this to help in family planning. If the couple want to have a baby then they should have sexual intercourse at this time. If the couple do not want to have a baby then they should avoid sexual intercourse at this time.

Using the correct names for different parts of the body should be encouraged, together with respect for the body and the words that we use. At first teachers and students may have problems with words like 'penis' and 'vagina', but these are the correct words and we need to learn to say them in the same way that we would say 'nose' or 'mouth'. Everyone has a nose and a mouth and everyone has a penis or a vagina, and we should feel equally comfortable using any of these words.

Many physical, social and emotional changes take place at puberty. Girls are usually more developed at the same age than boys, and since students in the class will be at different stages of development, it is important to emphasise that everyone is different and that there is a wide range of normal development. If there are students whose level of development in puberty is very different from most of their friends in the class, you may have to deal with this situation with some sensitivity and make sure that no student feels embarrassed or uncomfortable because of the words or actions of other students in the class.

Different types of behaviour relating to the human body can either promote or lessen respect. Examples of behaviour that can lessen respect are using names of body parts in an abusive way, touching someone in a sexual way and sexual harassment—giving attention to someone in a sexual way when the person does not want your attention.

Different types of behaviour can also promote growth and development; examples are diet, fitness and exercise, cleanliness and personal hygiene. Students should be able to find out about different situations, make decisions and take appropriate actions. Parents and teachers also have a responsibility to set a good example to young people by eating a balanced diet, not smoking and using alcohol in moderation.

Sexuality

Issues may arise due to the different rates of growth and development of young people. Adolescence can be a difficult and confusing time for some young people and for their parents and teachers, and students may need some help and guidance to describe these issues in their own adolescence. Students should be encouraged to express their feelings about each issue and to respect each other when they share their ideas openly. It is important to respect the ideas and feelings of others, and if students do not show respect at this time then teachers need to be ready to deal with the situation firmly and gently.

Different cultures have different beliefs about sexuality—the way we think and feel and behave as males or females. For example, some kinds of dressing, activities or behaviour are seen as being particularly masculine or feminine. Young children sometimes make fun of each other by saying that someone is a girl or boy when they are not, but most people grow out of this behaviour. From puberty onwards, adolescents become more aware of their sexual feelings and most people express their sexuality in the most satisfying way by eventually getting married, having sexual intercourse and being a parent. Sexual feelings are very strong in adolescence and students need to be aware of the consequences of their behaviour and ways of dealing with pressure from other people. Just because a person is capable of being a mother or a father does not mean that they are ready to be a husband or a wife and to take care of a baby. Students should be able to show responsibility in the way they deal with sexuality and in the decisions that they make.

The way that we behave towards other people can either encourage respect or reduce respect. Some examples of these types of behaviour are shown in the table below.

Behaviour that encourages respect	Behaviour that reduces respect
greeting someone by smiling and shaking hands	shouting or using bad language
being humble and not putting yourself above other people	interrupting other people and not letting them put their point of view
putting other people first by helping them	calling people names
comforting or caring for people who are old	being aggressive and wanting to fight
listening to different points of view	refusing to talk about important issues
accepting that there can be more than one correct answer or more than one way of doing something—not just your way	agreeing to do something then not doing it
being honest, reliable and trustworthy	being selfish and trying to get the best for yourself
being patient, reasonable and tolerant	criticising others either to their face or behind their back
being able to put yourself in somebody else's position and see things from his or her point of view	having many negative attitudes or making negative responses
showing generosity of spirit—accepting other people for who they are	not having time for other people
listening more than talking	repeating negative stories about other people
having a sense of humour even when things are difficult or go wrong	being unwilling to listen or to try to understand
facing and dealing with difficult situations	being unwilling to compromise

Nutrition

Nutrition is the study of food and the people that study food are called **nutritionists**. Nutrition also refers to the food that people eat and the way that their bodies use that food.

The basic nutrients or food groups are carbohydrates, fats, proteins, vitamins and fibre. Another way of classifying food is based on how the food is used by the body.

Food group	Nutrients (type of food)	Purpose or function
energy foods	carbohydrates and fats	provide energy for work and play, and warmth
growth foods	protein	for body building and repair
protective foods	vitamins and minerals	for protection from disease

Energy foods

Foods that contain carbohydrate and fat are energy foods, and carbohydrates can be divided into foods that contain starch and foods that contain sugar, as shown in the table below.

Carbohydrates		**Fats**
Starches	**Sugars**	
sweet potato taro yam cassava (tapioca) sago breadfruit corn banana rice bread biscuits	sugar sugar cane honey sweet fruits jam syrup	coconut cream margarine butter dripping oil—coconut oil, peanut oil, palm oil, pandanus oil breast milk

Protein foods

Protein foods can come from animals or from plants, as shown in the table below. Plant proteins are better for body building when different kinds are eaten at the same time.

Animal protein food	**Plant protein food**
meat—fresh and tinned fish—fresh and tinned shellfish crabs, prawns and crayfish birds insects—grubs and caterpillars snakes milk—powdered milk, tinned milk, breast milk eggs cheese	beans—winged beans, lima beans, soya beans, broad beans, mung beans, snake beans peas peanuts pandanus nuts other nuts, e.g. galip nuts coconut

Protective foods

Fresh fruits and vegetables containing vitamins and fibre are protective because they help the body to heal and repair itself.

Dark green leafy vegetables	**Red and yellow vegetables**
pumpkin tips aibika watercress ferns and other bush greens long and short pitpit green beans	tomatoes pumpkin carrots
Citrus fruits	**Red and yellow fruits**
oranges and mandarins (swit muli) lemons (muli) pomelo grapefruit	pawpaw guava mango pineapple

Planning meals using locally available food

When planning and preparing balanced meals, it is best to use food that is easily available in the local area, because it is more likely to be fresh and less expensive than food that comes from further away. It is important to remember that although growth foods usually come from animals, and therefore are more expensive, plants are also an important source of protein. The following table lists some examples of foods from the two main regions of Papua New Guinea.

Food group	Coastal food	Highlands food
energy foods that contain carbohydrates and fats	yam, taro, cassava, sago, sweet potato, potato, banana	sweet potato, English potato, pandanus oil
growth foods that contain protein	fish, shellfish, chicken, pork, eggs, peanuts, beans	chicken, pork, eggs, beans, winged beans, peanuts
protective foods that contain vitamins and minerals	aibika, pomelo, tomatoes, tulip	pumpkin tips, kumu, oranges, tomatoes

Since our health is affected by the food we eat, it is important to eat a balanced diet containing a mixture of foods from all food groups. Discuss with the students how it is possible to eat a balanced diet with foods that are available locally. Emphasise the importance of fresh foods that people can grow themselves or are grown or available in the local area, not expensive imported food. Emphasise the need to avoid foods that are high in fat or sugar or have extra salt added, all of which can cause health problems. These foods are sometimes called **fast foods** or **rubbish foods**.

Planning and preparing a nutritious meal that is suitable for the community using safe and hygienic methods is a useful and important skill for students to acquire. Again, actively encourage the use of healthy foods that are grown or are available in the local area, especially fruit and vegetables. Protein foods such as meat and fish are often expensive but protein can also be found in plant foods such as nuts and beans as well.

Food choices

Food choices are affected by such issues as availability, cost, the time taken in preparation and cultural beliefs. These influences explain why groups and individuals in the community may have different eating and meal patterns.

Health problems can be caused by not eating enough, or eating too much of, certain types of food. For example, Papua New Guinea has very high rates of malnutrition in children because they are not eating enough of the right kind of food, especially protein foods. As Papua New Guinea develops, new problems are appearing because of the food we eat—for example, tooth decay in children due to them having too many sweet foods and drinks. Becoming overweight is also becoming a health problem for some people, especially in urban areas, where a diet containing too much fat and sugar is made worse by not taking enough exercise and by smoking.

Suggested activities

Different strategies should be planned, developed and implemented to address a nutrition-related issue in the school. Examples are a school-lunch policy, a policy about the food that is available at the school canteen and the food that is given to visitors or is available on special occasions at the school, such as a concert or end-of-year ceremony.

Personal health and safety

There are a number of everyday behaviours that promote health, and we can all do certain things to keep ourselves clean, which will also help to keep us healthy. These are choices that people make and the responsibility is ours.

Common illnesses and diseases such as malaria, colds, gastroenteritis and grille are found in many communities but we know how they are spread from person to person. We can use this knowledge to protect ourselves, for example, by keeping ourselves and the community clean (or by following good hygiene) and by following simple rules about the way we use food and water, and the way we live together.

- **Common diseases in Papua New Guinea that cause death**
  - ➢ malaria
  - ➢ acute respiratory infection (ARI)
  - ➢ diarrhoea with dehydration
  - ➢ anaemia—usually due to malaria
  - ➢ meningitis
  - ➢ malnutrition
  - ➢ tuberculosis
  - ➢ alcohol causing road accidents
  - ➢ HIV/AIDS
- **Control of these diseases can be done through:**
  - ➢ treatment of common diseases
  - ➢ health promotion and education
  - ➢ immunisations
- **Diseases which can cause death that can be prevented by immunisations are:**
  - ➢ whooping cough
  - ➢ diphtheria
  - ➢ tetanus
  - ➢ poliomyelitis
  - ➢ pigbel
  - ➢ measles
  - ➢ tuberculosis
  - ➢ hepatitis B

Malaria

Malaria is carried by the *Anopheles* mosquito that bites at night. We can protect ourselves in the following ways:

- Get rid of breeding places for mosquitoes.
- Protect people from being bitten by mosquitoes by wearing long sleeves and long trousers at night; clearing away the bush from near houses and the places where water collects and mosquitoes lay eggs; and sleeping under bed nets treated with insecticide and sitting under a net that is big enough for the family.
- Give chloroquine once per week to people at greater risk of getting malaria: pregnant women and children living in malaria areas who have malnutrition, anaemia or a large spleen.

Other infections spread by mosquitoes are filariasis (elephantiasis) and dengue fever (breakbone fever). Dengue is spread by the *Aedes* mosquito that bites in the daytime.

Risks and hazards

Our health can also be affected by risks and hazards. A risk is a behaviour that can have a bad effect on our health or well-being and a hazard is a danger that we find in our surroundings.

There are many risks and hazards to our health and well-being at school, at home and in the community. We all need to think about risk assessment. This means we need to think about any possible bad effects on our health and safety because of the way that we behave. There are different levels of danger with each hazard. Some hazards have a high level of danger and some have a low level of danger. We need to understand the level of danger of each hazard. We need to know how we can reduce the danger because of the way that we behave.

Health goals

Health concerns will vary from community to community and from place to place, but there are some issues that affect some people in almost every community: the type and amount of food that people eat; smoking; drinking alcohol or taking other drugs; and sexually transmitted infections, including HIV/AIDS. Students should learn to develop health goals in relation to these concerns. The purpose is to get students to think about these issues before they are exposed to the risk, or before the issues have become a problem, so that they have a strategy or way of dealing with the situation. When a person is prepared for a particular situation, he or she is more likely to be able to deal with it in a satisfactory way. For example, being able to say no to any activity that is unhealthy or unsafe.

Students, like everyone else, are exposed to a variety of risks, and they need to develop their own way to deal with these. They need to understand the possible outcomes from their behaviour and take responsibility for themselves. For example, sexually transmitted infections including HIV/AIDS are a serious problem in Papua New Guinea. Some health experts believe that the country is beginning to suffer an epidemic similar to that which has occurred in countries in Africa and Asia, where hundreds of thousands of people have been killed by the disease. In some African countries, grandparents are trying to look after young children and work in the garden because most of the productive adults who normally produce the food and take care of children have died from AIDS. The impact of AIDS on life expectancy in a number of countries is shown in the *Papua New Guinea Primary School Atlas* (page 51). Although some communities may find it difficult to talk about sexually transmitted infections, teachers have a responsibility to make students aware of the possible result of their behaviour and help them to develop the skills and attitudes that allow them to deal with the situation. Some people may feel uncomfortable talking about HIV/AIDS, but dying from AIDS due to lack of information may be the alternative.

HIV/AIDS

Acquired Immune Deficiency Syndrome, or AIDS, is caused by the virus known as the Human Immunodeficiency Virus, or HIV. When the HIV virus enters the body it is attracted to particular cells of the immune system in blood, semen and vaginal fluid.

HIV carriers are infectious but look and feel well. HIV is spread by:

- sexual intercourse with an infected partner
- infected instruments like needles or knives
- infected mother to unborn child

The HIV virus is not spread by food, water, insects or toilet seats. It is not spread by everyday contact such as shaking hands, living together, playing together, eating together and hugging—provided there is no body contact with the wounds or body fluids of one person to another.

Signs and symptoms of AIDS

In the first stage people may have the following: fever, enlarged glands, night sweats, headache and cough. However, many people who are infected with HIV have none of these.

In the second stage, or carrier stage, people feel well and have no symptoms.

The third stage is fully developed HIV infection and it may take many years to reach this stage. The HIV virus has broken down the immunity of the body so that the patient easily gets infections and cancers. The main symptoms and signs include weight loss of more than 10 per cent in adults, chronic diarrhoea for more than one month, and prolonged fever for more than one month. The minor symptoms and signs can be many but may include swollen glands and repeated common infections.

Caring for people with AIDS in the home

There is no cure for AIDS. In some countries drugs are available to help the patient, but they are very expensive and are not normally available in Papua New Guinea. Patients should be treated to ease the symptoms of the disease.

People with AIDS also suffer from the fear of death and are worried about the problems that may arise in the future. They may also feel rejected and isolated by the rest of the community. People with AIDS need the care and support of the people around them. They can be cared for in the home and there is little danger to other people provided the following guidelines are followed:

- People with AIDS do not need to have their own saucepans, plates, cups and spoons, but these things should be washed properly with soapy water in the normal way (hot water is best).
- People with AIDS should have their own bed sheets, towel, toothbrush and shaving equipment and should not share these with anyone else.
- Bed sheets, towels and clothes that are lightly soiled with saliva, urine, sweat or vomit should be washed in soapy water in the normal way (hot water is best). All laundry should be hung outside in the sun to dry.
- Bed sheets, towels and clothes that are heavily soiled with blood, large amounts of vomit or diarrhoea should not be touched directly. Wear gloves or use towels or paper to cover them or lift them with a stick or bamboo tongs like carrying hot mumu stones. Wash the items in plenty of cold running water and then soak in water containing disinfectant for one hour or boil the items in a copper for at least twenty minutes. All laundry should be hung outside in the sun to dry.
- Clean floors by removing blood or vomit with paper while wearing gloves. Wash with soapy water and then wipe over with disinfectant.

Safety

There are many causes and effects of behaviour that affect our safety in the community. For example, drinking has become a big social and health problem in many places. Drinking too much can end in fighting and violence, which can injure people and damage property. Drinking and driving is also the cause of motor vehicle accidents that injure or kill people. Teachers, parents and others in the community need to set a good example to young people in their drinking behaviour.

Rape has also become an important issue, particularly for girls and women in many parts of Papua New Guinea. Students need to learn the importance of respecting the rights of all people to feel safe. Communities need to develop a sense of trust and responsibility and to deal with offenders in ways that are appropriate.

A number of health issues are of concern to young people. For example, young people often want to appear grown up and see smoking as adult behaviour, so they smoke as a way of trying to show they are mature. Unfortunately, they are copying a foolish adult behaviour and in the process may become addicted to tobacco, a habit that is hard to break and which creates more health problems than any other single cause.

There is often pressure on young people to dress, behave and think in certain ways and to listen to certain types of music. This is sometimes called 'peer group pressure' or 'peer pressure'. Most young people want to feel that they belong to a group and the need to conform and be accepted by the group can be strong. Young people need to be encouraged to make careful choices about the friends they spend time with, and teachers and parents need to be sensitive about the way they deal with situations like this.

Safe sexual behaviour and sexual responsibilities are also important. Depending on their experience and personality, and the way that students respond, some teachers will find this a challenging topic to deal with. Think about the ways that you can provide information to students and the way you will deal with questions and discussion. Providing written information can sometimes be easier for people who find it difficult to talk about sexuality. If students are reluctant to ask questions, or if you would like time to think about your response to a question, students can write questions on pieces of paper without their name and put them in a box. You can then take them away and look at the questions, think about the answers and check information if needed. Next lesson you can bring the questions into the class, pull out a question at a time and answer them. If students are reluctant to discuss sexuality, or to ask questions in mixed groups, you can organise single sex groups.

The ethical values of dignity, self-respect and respect for others, along with respect for the values of the community, should be encouraged.

Finally, students should be encouraged to develop ways to deal with unsafe or risky situations. Students should learn how to use equipment properly and how to take precautions and follow the rules in relation to road safety, fire and water safety, using tools and so on. When faced with an unexpected situation, encourage students to learn to rely on their instinct or gut feeling. If something does not feel 'quite right' then it probably isn't, and it may be safer to get out of that situation. They should alert others and try to make the situation safer without putting themselves in more danger. If someone else is in danger, we should try to help that person if it is safe to do so.

Community health

Community health includes the most important health concerns in the community and ways of caring for the community in order to promote health. Major health concerns vary from place to place but are likely to include malnutrition, malaria and sexually transmitted infections.

Malnutrition—or failure to grow properly

- People can have malnutrition when they don't eat enough of the right kind of food, don't eat enough food or eat too much food. Malnutrition is very common in Papua New Guinea and malnourished children are always underweight, get infections easily and die more easily than other children. Malnutrition usually occurs because people do not eat enough of the right kind of food. This includes all kinds of food—energy foods and protein or growth foods. Because of this it is sometimes called *Protein Energy Malnutrition* or PEM. Some children suffer from malnutrition and infections at the same time. Malnutrition makes infections worse and infections make malnutrition worse.

Marasmus (starvation)

- Children get marasmus because they eat too little food of any kind and so they are very underweight and look very thin ('skin and bone'). They may also have diarrhoea and anaemia.

Kwashiorkor

- Kwashiorkor is an African word that means 'the disease that occurs when the child is pushed away from the breast because of another child'. Children get kwashiorkor when they don't eat enough protein. A child with kwashiorkor may look fat, but when you feel the arms and legs the muscles are thin. They may also have diarrhoea and there may be changes in their hair and skin.

Common causes of malnutrition	Treatment
not enough food	give more food, more often
many children in family	family planning
problems in the family or house	educate for change in family living or environment

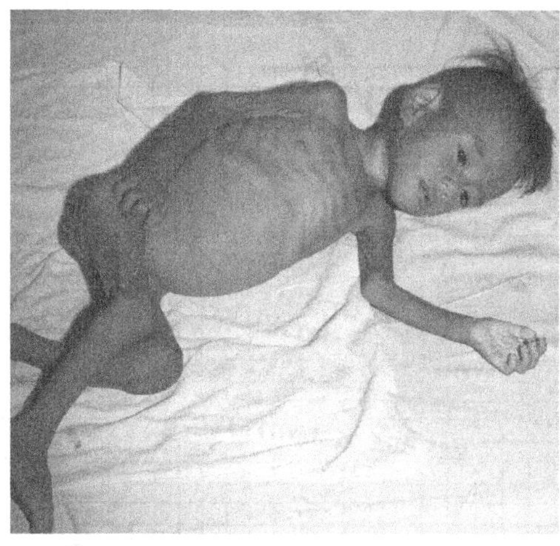
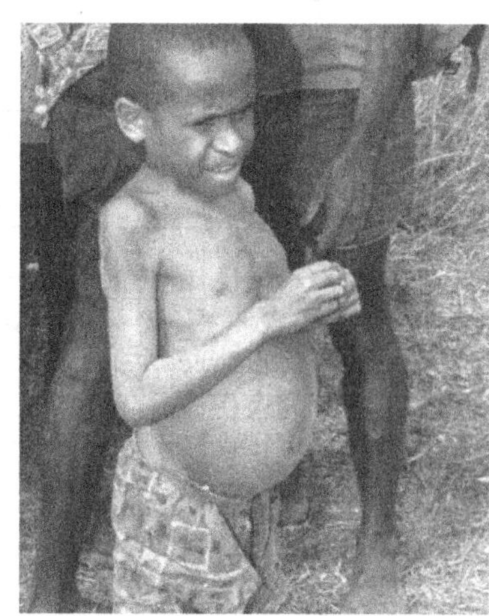

Figure 5.1 A child with marasmus and a child with kwashiorkor.

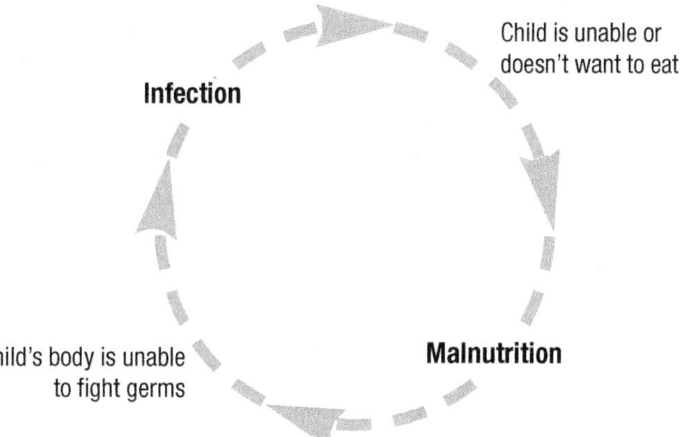

Figure 5.2 Circle of infection and malnutrition. Malnutrition makes infections worse and infections make malnutrition worse

Source: Smith, Dr Clifford (1996) *Health Care Manual for Community Health Workers, 2e*, page 282.

RULES FOR GOOD NUTRITION IN CHILDREN

1 Breast feed for as long as possible (at least eighteen months). Breast milk is best for babies.

2 Start solid foods at four months (or if age is not known, as soon as first tooth appears). Mash up a staple food to make a porridge.

3 Add high energy foods to the staple porridge—feed children a spoonful of dripping or other oil by adding it to the porridge.

4 Add protein foods to the staple porridge—give cooked and ground up peanuts, beans or fish every day.

5 Add protective foods to the staple porridge—add some yellow, orange and green foods each day.

6 Give at least four to six meals a day to children. Give the food meal each time before the breast milk.

7 Give food as often as possible to sick children.

A child should be eating a balanced meal by the age of six months.

We can keep a check on the health of children by measuring their weight regularly. Children who are fed properly and who are not sick repeatedly will put on weight steadily and follow a good 'road to health' as shown in the graph:

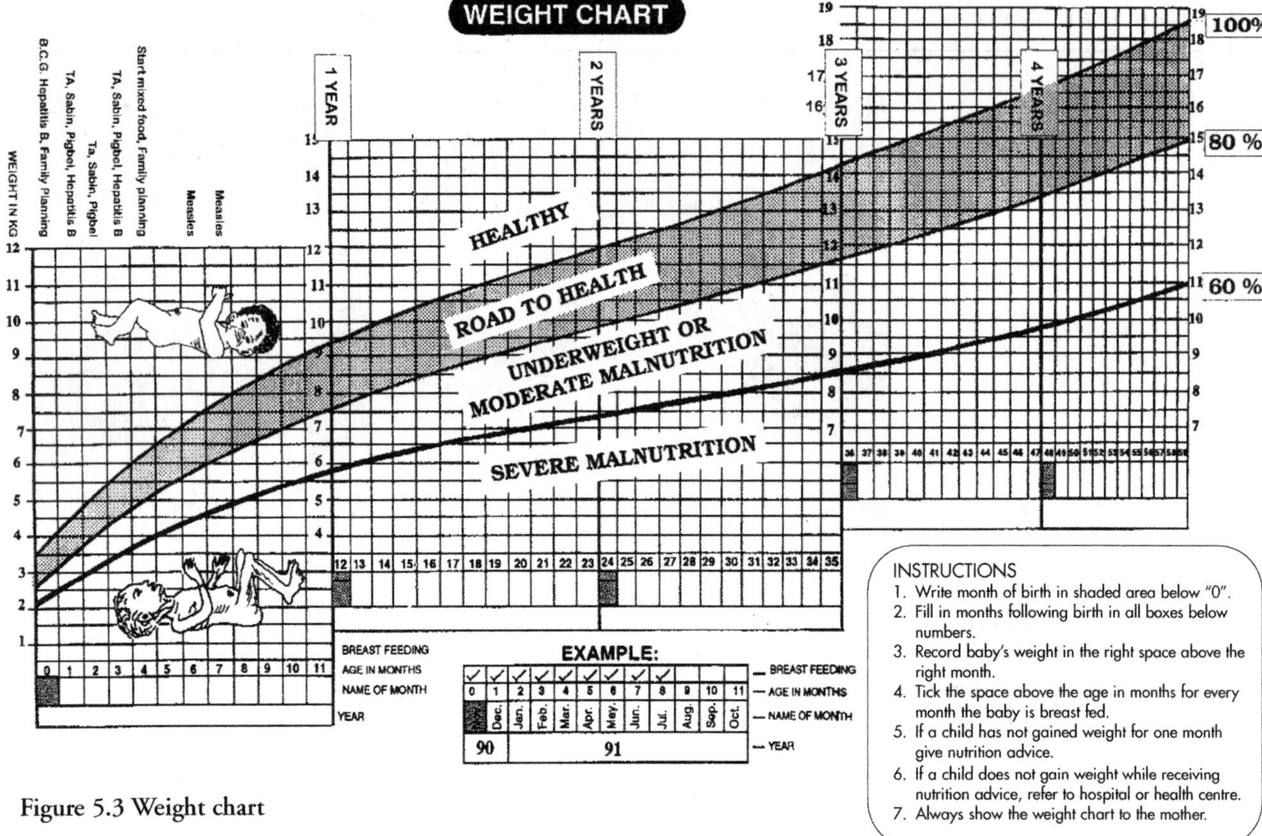

Figure 5.3 Weight chart

Health Services

Due to economic problems in Papua New Guinea, health services to rural areas have reduced in recent years. In some provinces, aid posts have closed and there is a general shortage of medicines. This means that in some places it is impossible to get treatment. You will therefore need to adapt this part of the topic on Health Services according to the situation in your area. What alternative ways have people found to deal with this situation?

Health promotion

'Health promotion' means all the activities that we do in order to help people to stay healthy in the community. This includes health education, which doesn't only happen in schools but through radio and television awareness programs and advertisements. Health promotion also includes immunisation programs to prevent diseases, spraying or fogging against mosquitoes, and improving housing, food and water supplies and sanitation (rubbish collection and sewerage). Health promotion activities can be provided by the Department of Health, by Local Level Government Councils (LLGs) and by town councils, but people in the community can also carry out activities to promote the health of their community. The community are the *stakeholders* in health promotion because they have a *stake,* or particular interest, in the activities and the results or outcomes of the activities.

Health promotion activities should be planned and carried out with the involvement or participation of the stakeholders. For example, when planning an improvement to a water supply the community must be involved in the planning of the project and can also help in the work of the project. In many communities women and girls do most of the work in carrying water and their voice should be heard. By encouraging equal participation and decision-making from men and women, the project will be more likely to meet the needs of the community, and they will feel ownership of the project and work towards maintaining it.

Human behaviour is having an increasing effect on the environment and this in turn can affect our health. Examples from different communities in Papua New Guinea include waste disposal, logging, mining, and emissions from industry and vehicles that pollute the air, land and water. How are these having an effect on the way that people live, including their health? You may not be able to do much about big problems, but we can all do something about the way that we dispose of our own rubbish at school and at home. Encourage students to be responsible at school and in their home communities. This should become a habit, or good practice, that we follow every day, not just something that we do from time to time or when we have a clean-up campaign.

Amongst community health concerns, one of the greatest dangers is from chemicals that are released into the environment which then get taken in by animals when they eat and drink. Bigger animals (or carnivores) eat smaller animals, which has the effect of increasing, concentrating or multiplying the chemicals further along the food chain. When humans eat animals they may be taking in chemicals or poisons that came from the plants that were eaten by the first animal (in this case, a herbivore) in the food chain. Encourage students to find ways to minimise or prevent these health concerns and to gather the relevant information before making informed decisions about healthy living.

The increase in the size of the population is having a noticeable effect on the provision of health services and community facilities. In the thirty years since independence in 1975, the size of the population has grown from about three million to about five million people. Traditionally, people in Papua New Guinea had big families and there are both positive and negative effects of a large family size. Government departments like the Department of Education and the Department of Health have never been able to provide sufficient services to all the people, and this has become more difficult as the population has rapidly increased, especially at a time when Papua New Guinea is having economic difficulties. Finding enough money for food, clothing, transport and school fees is difficult for many people. Parents now must think carefully about the number of children they will have. Family planning allows parents to decide the number and spacing of their children.

Selected social indicators, such as the percentage of malnourished children under five and the percentage of the population with access to clean water, can be used to compare the situation of Papua New Guinea with other countries (refer to the *Papua New Guinea Primary School Atlas*, page 51).

Drugs

Use of drugs

People use a variety of drugs in a number of different ways. We can classify all drugs into a number of groups, depending on the way they are used and controlled.

Medicines include everyday drugs like painkillers and cough medicines that we can obtain from the store without a prescription from a doctor. They also include prescription drugs that we get from the hospital pharmacy or pharmacy store after seeing a doctor. Medicines can be used for the prevention, diagnosis and treatment of disease. Other drugs like caffeine, which is found in tea, coffee and cola drinks, are legal and not harmful. However, some drugs are legal but can be harmful, such as tobacco and alcohol and betel nut chewed with lime. Finally, some drugs are illegal and all of these can be harmful.

The different types of drugs that people use can be summarised in a table:

Categories of drugs

Medicines		Other drugs—legal		Other drugs—illegal
Non-prescription	**Prescription**	**Harmless (in small quantities)**	**Harmful**	
analgesics (e.g. Panadol, paracetamol, aspirin)	antibiotics—against bacteria	tea	tobacco	cannabis, marijuana
Cough medicine	antimalarials (e.g. quinine)	coffee	betel nut chewed with lime	amphetamines
	antihistaminzes—to treat allergies	cola drinks	alcohol (if too much is drunk)	heroin
	sedatives—to calm people		methylated spirit	cocaine
	anaesthetics—to stop people feeling pain			

People use drugs for different reasons. Some of these uses are beneficial since they prevent or cure illness, but some are harmful—even though the drug may make the person feel good when they are taking it. Drugs that are used to feel good are sometimes called 'recreational drugs'.

Why people use drugs

There are many factors that affect the decisions people make about whether or not to take drugs. Students should be able to gather information about the consequences of taking drugs, analyse the information and make wise decisions. Students should learn about the ways they can respond when people put pressure on them or try to force them to use drugs that are harmful. Students should work out different strategies or ways of doing this and practise saying no to drugs in different situations. You can use role plays to get the students to practise these skills.

Commonly used drugs

Drug use has a number of effects in the community including the breakdown in law and order and relationships. Cigarettes and alcohol are two drugs that are commonly used in Papua New Guinea and both cause health problems. Smoking has short- and long-term effects that can affect both the smoker and people close to the smoker through passive smoking, which occurs when people breathe in the air that contains smoke. Smoking is the single largest cause of preventable disease in the world and this is expected to continue into the future. Getting people to stop smoking would prevent more disease than any other health intervention that we could use. Unfortunately, governments earn large amounts of money from the tax or duty on tobacco, so they are often reluctant to introduce policies or laws that will reduce the amount of tobacco that is sold.

Tobacco

Smoking is one of the biggest health problems in the world. When people smoke for a long time, then there can be serious effects on their health. Tobacco contains a drug called nicotine, which means that tobacco is habit-forming or can cause an addiction. Once people start smoking they often find it very hard to stop, even when they understand that it can cause health problems. Many smokers begin when they are young and later find that they cannot give up. For these reasons it is best to never start smoking, and young people need to be encouraged never to start smoking. Young people should never be offered cigarettes and should not be allowed to buy cigarettes. Teachers should be good role models and should not smoke. Nobody should smoke in a building so that other people have to breathe in air that contains tobacco smoke. Women who are pregnant should not smoke because smoking can harm the baby.

Ways to stop smoking

Although it may not be easy for someone who has been smoking for a long time to stop, the following may help:

- List the benefits of stopping smoking.
- Note the times of the day when you are more likely to smoke and the things that make you want to smoke. Think of other things that you can do at this time, using your hands or putting something in your mouth instead of lighting a cigarette. Write these alternatives down as a plan so that you will be prepared.
- Set a date when you will stop smoking. A good time is when there is some other important change in your life.

It takes three or four days for the nicotine to get out of the bloodstream and this is the hardest time. It then takes between four and six weeks for the body to get used to the change. People need encouragement and support during this time.

Reasons why people smoke	Disadvantages of smoking
It gives pleasure It settles nerves It boosts confidence It provides a 'lift' and makes people feel better People smoke when they have a drink People smoke after they have eaten a meal	It reduces fitness It stains teeth It makes breath and clothes smell It puts people at risk of diseases such as cancer and emphysema It makes people cough It costs a lot of money

Diseases caused by smoking
cancers—lung, mouth, larynx, stomach, bladder, breast
other lung diseases—bronchitis and emphysema
other inflammations—laryngitis (larynx and vocal cords), sinusitis
narrowing of the arteries causing heart disease and strokes
thinning of the bones—osteoporosis
problems in pregnancy—miscarriage, slower growth of babies

Alcohol

Alcohol is absorbed directly from the stomach and affects the brain. However, alcohol does not get into the bloodstream and to the brain as quickly if there is food in the stomach.

The table below shows the possible effects of drinking by an average-sized man; women generally get drunk more quickly.

Stage	Number of drinks (in one hour)*	Behaviour
Feeling relaxed	3–5 bottles of beer	talks a lot, concentrates less, unsafe to drive
Acts like a 'big head' (danger state)	6–9 bottles of beer	fighting doing things that the person is ashamed of later
Drunk (harmful state)	0–20 bottles of beer 1–2 bottles of wine or $\frac{1}{2}$ bottle of spirits	slow speech poor balance blurred eyesight vomiting needs help walking falls asleep
Drunken stupor	30–40 bottles of beer $1\frac{1}{2}$ bottles of spirits	breathes heavily no bladder control unconscious
Death	More than the above	None

* Although the time mentioned in the table is one hour, drinking a large quantity of alcohol over several hours is also dangerous and can make people drunk.

People who drink too much alcohol over many years often develop health problems such as alcoholism, cirrhosis of the liver, cancer, brain damage and malnutrition. Drinking can become dangerous or harmful when we drink too much, especially for people who drink regularly. Drinking a lot in a short period of time is also dangerous even if people only do this occasionally. This is called 'binge drinking'. There is also an important difference between drinking in men and women. Because their bodies are different, women can drink less than men before it becomes harmful or dangerous, as shown in the two tables below:

Standard drinks per day*

	Low risk	Dangerous	Harmful
Male	less than 4	5–6	more than 6
Female	less than 2	3–4	more than 4

Standard drinks per week*

	Low risk	Dangerous	Harmful
Male	less than 28	28–42	more than 42
Female	less than 14	14–28	more than 28

* When drinks are bought by the bottle or can, they are not standard drinks. One bottle or can of beer is the same as one-and-a-half standard drinks.

Alcohol affects behaviour and has become a social problem as well as being a health problem. Heavy drinkers can be violent and want to fight. Spending money on alcohol also means that there is not always enough money for important things like food, clothing and school fees. Again, teachers and other adults in the community are role models for young people and should set a good example for students to follow. If you drink, then drink in moderation and never get drunk or lose control of your drinking and behaviour.

Betel nut

Although betel nut is important on social occasions in many parts of Papua New Guinea, there are health effects associated with using betel nut, especially when it is chewed with lime, which is usually the case.

Betel nut is acidic and the lime is used to neutralise the acid which improves the taste in the mouth. Unfortunately, this combination can lead to cancer of the mouth, tongue or cheeks (due to a chemical called a carcinogen). The cancer usually begins as a small spot or sore, but it can grow large if the person continues to chew betel nut. In severe cases the cheek of the person may be completely eaten away, leaving a hole.

For these reasons, it is best not to chew betel nut, and anyone who has a sore or a spot should stop chewing and visit a health worker.

Marijuana

Marijuana is another drug that is grown and used in Papua New Guinea. Since people smoke this drug it can lead to lung disease and respiratory illness. People who use marijuana for a long time can also develop mental or psychiatric problems and may find that it is difficult to lead a normal life.

People in the community who have developed the habit of taking drugs that are harmful, so that this has become a problem, need the understanding and support of the community. There are few agencies or organisations in Papua New Guinea that can help people with drug problems and these are likely to be in urban areas, but church groups and families can support people who are using harmful drugs.

The effects of drugs

The effects of producing, selling or using drugs can be positive or negative and some of these effects are listed in the table below.

Effect of producing, selling or using drugs	Positive effect	Negative effect
Smoking can lead to diseases such as lung cancer and liver disease		✓
Farmers earn money from growing and selling tobacco	✓	
Drinking can cause accidents, such as road accidents, and death		✓
Provincial governments earn money from the tax on beer	✓	
Drinking and drug use can cause family violence and abuse		✓
Drinking and drug use can lead to family breakdown		✓
Drinking and drug can cause crime as people steal to pay for drugs		✓
National government earns money from the tax on tobacco	✓	

STRAND 5

Living and Working Together

About this strand

This strand introduces the main ideas and behaviour that are the foundation for people living and working together harmoniously in the community. The decisions and choices that people make about the way they live are based on ethical values. There are different influences on our decision-making, and following steps in this process can reduce the negative results that can come from poor decisions. A good leader should possess a set of desirable qualities that can be used when we want to choose a leader. We all have expectations of a leader, and elected leaders should be chosen, and changed, using a system that is fair. Rules and laws are underpinned by values and help people to live happily and safely; there are consequences of upholding and breaking them. Similarly, our rights and freedom of expression, movement and lifestyle are based on common standards of acceptable behaviour.

Sub-strands 1–4

Main ideas

Sub-strand 1: People make choices in the way they live together; their decisions are based on ethical values and can have positive and negative results.

Sub-strand 2: Good and fair leaders have certain qualities, which can be used to choose who will be a leader. People have expectations of leaders.

Sub-strand 3: Communities have rules and laws for safety and protection and we all have a duty and obligation to uphold laws so that we can live in harmony.

Sub-strand 4: There are community standards of behaviour that support rights and freedoms.

Key words

Choices, decision-making, community service, ethical values, rules, laws, duties, obligations, rights, freedoms, leadership, elections, discrimination

Assessment tasks

Assessment aims to gather information on how well students have achieved the outcomes of the Living and Working Together strand. A variety of strategies should be used: written, oral and practical.

Each assessment item should be based on criteria that have been clearly written down. Students should be told what the criteria are so that they know the basis for judgment of their achievement and demonstration of the outcomes. In this way teachers will be able to measure how well the students have achieved the learning outcomes. Teachers should focus on the performance of each individual and be much less interested in comparing the performance of one student against another.

Assessment should also be continuous and collected throughout the learning process by the completion of appropriate activities such as those indicated with the assessment icon in the 'For you to try' sections.

Major links to other subjects

Living and Working Together links to the substrands 'cultural expression' and 'societies and communities' of Social Science, and the substrand 'knowing your community' and 'communication' of Making a Living. Aspects of different subjects can be integrated into activities such as:

- a health project to care for our body
- collecting and analysing statistical data for specific diseases
- designing posters to relay the message of healthy living.
- reading and planning recipes
- measuring ingredients for specific purposes
- designing healthy eating plans

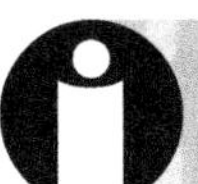

Teacher information

Making choices

The decisions people make are usually based on their ethical values—the things they say or believe are important. Some groups or organisations have a code of ethics that tells people how to behave and reminds members of their responsibilities. For example, teachers in Papua New Guinea are guided by the PNG Teachers' Association Code of Ethics.

PAPUA NEW GUINEA TEACHERS' ASSOCIATION CODE OF ETHICS

Teaching is a profession. Membership of a profession carries with it obligations as well as privileges. These obligations concern loyalty, discipline, justice and service to the community. It is essential to create a body of teachers who conform to recognised ethics, who conduct themselves honourably in their professional practice, and who do their utmost to promote and maintain the dignity and welfare of the teaching service and their profession as a whole.

A. RESPONSIBILITY TO THE CHILD

Professional teachers desire their pupils to attain the highest level of mental, moral and physical health and development. They therefore:

1. *set an example in behaviour, dress and appearance acceptable to the community*
2. *work to instil into the child respect for elders and for cultural differences*
3. *aim to develop self-reliance, self-development and self-discipline in the children, being always mindful of the differences in their needs and abilities*
4. *strive to prepare their pupils to take their place as citizens who are concerned with the welfare of the community and the nation*

B. RESPONSIBILITY TO THE COMMUNITY AND THE NATION

The professional teacher adopts a friendly, cooperative and constructive relationship with the community and works therein to advance the cause of education. They:

1. *respect the community they serve and are willing to participate in community activities*
2. *encourage cooperation and understanding between teachers and parents, school and community*
3. *strive to keep themselves informed on matters of community and national importance*

C. RESPONSIBILITY TO THE PROFESSION

As a member of a profession teachers should be committed to striving for the highest level of personal integrity, professional competence and academic achievement for their own betterment and that of the profession as a whole. They:

1. *adopt high standards of integrity and loyalty which create mutual respect between teachers and adds distinction to the profession*
2. *exercise discretion in dealing with matters relating to the pupil, the pupil's parents and their fellow teachers*
3. *are constructive in their criticism of staff, school and students*
4. *improve the quality of their own teaching and continually expand their own knowledge by keeping up with educational trends*
5. *maintain an active membership in a professional association of teachers as a means of achieving betterment of the profession and education as a whole*
6. *do not use their social, civic or professional activities to obtain favour or preferment of their profession*

D. RESPONSIBILITY TO THE EMPLOYER AND THE AGENCY

The professional teachers' fulfilment of their obligations to employer and agency is based on respect for lawful authority and the need for mutual cooperation. They:

1. *acquaint themselves with current terms and conditions of their employment*
2. *obey the rules and regulations of the employer in principle and practice as well as the philosophy of the agency*
3. *have regard for the accepted process of appeal, conciliation and arbitration as a means of challenging rules and regulations or their interpretation*
4. *show initiative in the fulfilment of their duties*
5. *refrain from any activity detrimental to the effectiveness of their professional responsibilities*

Learning how to make good choices and decisions is an essential skill we use every day. Making decisions about important things that happen in our lives can be quite difficult. It helps to have a method or consistent approach in order to help make decisions. Each step must be completed before moving on to the next. It can be very helpful to write down the answers to these questions because writing something down makes you think more carefully, and then you can compare the possible results from different choices.

Steps in the decision-making process

1 What is the *issue* or the *problem*?

2 What are the *options* or *choices* you can make?

3 What are the *good things* and the *bad things* that can happen as a result of *each* option?

4 Make your decision after thinking about the *possibilities*.

5 How do you *feel* about the choices you have made?

After making your decision and seeing the result, the last step is to think about the decision and decide if it was a good one. This is known as 'evaluating the outcome'. If your decision was a good one, then you will probably feel more confident about making decisions in the future. If your decision was a bad one, then you need to try to find out why it was not a good decision so that you do not make the same mistake again.

Making choices—classroom or school issues

In recent years people have begun to notice new problems in schools and in the community which show that people do not care for the environment or surroundings or show respect to people:

- **Vandalism**—deliberately trying to damage or spoil buildings or things that belong to other people or to the community. In some cases people may also deliberately set fire to buildings, which is called 'arson'.
- **Graffiti**—using paint to write names or make other signs and symbols on walls and buildings.
- **Littering**—dropping rubbish anywhere instead of putting it in a rubbish bin.
- **Harassment and abuse**—annoying or aggravating people and treating them with cruelty and violence.

Vandalism, graffiti and littering all make the community less attractive and a less pleasant place to live. These things give the feeling that people do not care, and this may discourage other people from being responsible in their behaviour. On the other hand, when the environment is clean and attractive, people may be more encouraged to try to keep it that way.

When we live in a community, or when we visit a community, then we get an impression of the way that people live and the way that they treat each other and the surroundings. The choices that they make, and the effects of their choices will be clear. When people make good choices based on ethical values then the community is likely be a safe, clean and pleasant place in which people respect each other and live in harmony.

Sexual violence and abuse

Papua New Guinea has new, tougher laws on sexual violence and abuse. These laws give more protection to victims (both male and female) and have higher penalties for offenders. The Criminal Code on Sexual Offences and the Evidence Act, which contains the above laws, were gazetted on 10 April 2003.

If you, or someone you know, has been a victim of these crimes you should contact the police, your local church or women's organisations.

The following laws apply to non-consenting sexual activity involving men or women over sixteen years old:

Rape

- It is a crime to force sex on a man or a woman.
- It is a crime to put a penis into another person's mouth without their consent.
- It is a crime to put any body part (finger etc.) into another person's anus or vagina without their consent.
- It is a crime to put any object (stick, bottle etc.) into another person's anus or vagina without their consent.
- It is a crime for a man to force his wife to have sex against her will.

Punishment: Jail for up to fifteen years. If the crime is especially bad (pack rape, with weapons etc.) the guilty person can be jailed for life.

Sexual assault

- It is a crime to touch the sexual parts of another person's body without their consent.
- It is a crime to make someone touch the sexual parts of another person.

Punishment: Jail for up to five years. If the crime is especially bad the guilty person can be jailed for up to ten years.

Procuring a sexual offence

- It is a crime to order a sexual attack on another person. For example, a person who orders a pay-back rape is guilty of a crime even if they did not actually do the rape themselves.

Punishment: Jail for up to twenty years.

Sex crimes against children

These crimes apply to any sexual activity (consenting or not) with a boy or girl under the age of sixteen:

Sexual penetration of children

- It is a crime to have sex with a child, boy or girl.
- It is a crime to put a penis into a child's mouth.
- It is a crime to put any body part (finger etc.) into a child's anus or vagina.
- It is a crime to put any object (stick, bottle etc.) into a child's anus or vagina.

Punishment: Jail for up to twenty-five years. But if the victim is under twelve years old, or the guilty person has abused a position of trust (teacher, wantok, religious leader etc.), he or she can be jailed for life.

Sexual touching of a child

- It is a crime to touch a child in a sexual way.
- It is a crime to force a child to touch anyone else in a sexual way.

Punishment: Jail for up to seven years. But if the victim is under twelve years old, or the guilty person has abused a position of trust, he or she can be jailed for up to twelve years.

Indecent act directed at a child

- It is a crime to expose oneself to a child in a sexual way.
- It is a crime to make children expose themselves in a sexual way.

Punishment: Jail for up to five years. But if the victim is under twelve years old, or the guilty person has abused a position of trust, he or she can be jailed for up to seven years.

Persistent sexual abuse of a child

- It is a crime to commit any of these sex crimes against children over a long period of time.

Punishment: Jail for up to fifteen years.

Abuse of trust, authority or dependency.

It is legal to have consenting sex with a child over sixteen, except in the following cases:

- It is a crime for people in a position of trust or authority (teachers, religious instructors, adoptive parents, police officers etc.) to have any consenting sexual relationship with a child aged sixteen to eighteen years old who is in their care.
- If there is no consent, the crime is rape.

Punishment: Jail for up to fifteen years.

Child prostitution and child pornography

Child prostitution and child pornography are unacceptable in Papua New Guinea. The new laws punish all people who make children do these things.

Child prostitution is buying or selling sexual acts with a boy or girl under eighteen years old, in return for money, goods or favours (payment of school fees etc.)

- It is a crime to use a child as a prostitute or to offer to buy a child prostitute's services.
- It is a crime to let your home or place be used for child prostitution.
- It is a crime to get any benefits from child prostitution.
- It is a crime for a parent to let a child be used in child prostitution.
- It is not a crime for a child to be a prostitute. Child prostitutes are victims, not criminals.

Punishment: Jail for up to life, in some cases.

Child pornography is pictures and films that show children under eighteen years old doing sexual things. Sometimes it can also be audiotapes and writings.

- It is a crime to make or publish child pornography.
- It is a crime to import, export, distribute, sell or display child pornography.
- It is a crime to have child pornography in your home or bag.
- It is a crime to get a child for, or let your child make pornography.

Punishment: Jail for up to fifteen years, in some cases.

Giving evidence in court

The evidence laws introduced in 2003 try to make it easier for victims of sex crimes to tell their story. For example:

- You do not need evidence or another witness to prove your case. The court can convict on your evidence alone.
- The police are not allowed to tell the accused where you live.

There are also many rules to make being in court less scary. For example:

- The judge can tell the public to leave the court when you give your evidence.
- You can have a support person with you while you testify.
- The accused person is not allowed to cross-examine you.

Limited Preferential Voting

Elections for the National Parliament of Papua New Guinea, including by-elections, now use the Limited Preferential Voting (LPV) system.

The ballot paper contains the names and photographs of the candidates who are standing for election with a box next to each for the voter to show his or her choice. The voter must make three choices from the candidates listed on the ballot paper using the numbers 1, 2 and 3. The number 1 is used to indicate the voter's first choice or most preferred candidate. The number 2 is used to indicate the voter's second choice or second preferred candidate. The number 3 is used to indicate the third choice or third preferred candidate. No other marks should be placed on the ballot paper. If a voter puts other marks on the ballot paper it will not be counted.

For a candidate to be elected under this system, he or she must receive more than half, or 50 per cent, of the formal votes cast in the election. The number of formal votes that make up more than half is called an 'absolute majority' because once a candidate has reached this number of votes no other candidate can obtain a greater number of votes.

For example, if 1000 votes have been counted in a ballot, a candidate must get more than 500 votes to win.

First, all the number ones, or the voters' first choices, are distributed and then counted. If one candidate has an absolute majority, which means they get more than half the votes counted, then that person is the winner.

If no one has reached an absolute majority, the next step is to eliminate the candidate who got the smallest number of votes. The second choices shown on this candidate's ballot papers are now counted by distributing them to the remaining candidates and adding to their first votes.

If one candidate now has an absolute majority, or more than half the votes counted, then that person is the winner. Once again, if no one has reached an absolute majority, the next candidate who has the least number of votes is eliminated and the choices on this candidate's ballot papers are distributed to the remaining candidates and added to their previous votes. If there are any votes here from the first candidate to be eliminated, the third choices are now counted.

If one candidate now has an absolute majority or more than half the votes counted then that person is the winner. If not, this distribution of preferences continues until one candidate wins with an absolute majority.

The rule of law

Rules and laws show people the way that they should behave and make it easier for people to live together in the community. There are benefits and sometimes rewards for people who follow rules and laws, and there are punishments for people who break rules and laws, depending on the circumstances.

Consequences of breaking rules and laws

Setting	Consequences
Family	Parents or other adults will tell children when they break family rules. Privileges may be withdrawn or other punishments given. For example, parents may stop children doing something that they really enjoy doing or may set rules about where children can go or who they can meet.
School	Teachers will discipline children when they break school rules. Privileges may be withdrawn. Some teachers may punish children. For more serious rules, a student may be suspended so that they are not allowed to attend classes for a time or the student may be expelled from the school. Serious cases need to be decided by the Board of Management and endorsed by the Provincial Education Board.
Village	Village people may criticise, refuse to cooperate with or ignore those who repeatedly break the rules of the community. Some communities have their own village court that can make decisions about the lower levels of rules or laws that may have been broken.
Nation	Depending on the crime and the law that has been broken, the police may bring the person to the District Court, National Court or Supreme Court and the case will be decided by a magistrate or a judge. Depending on the crime, the punishment can include a fine or being sent to a corrective institute for many months or years. People with a criminal record may not be able to hold certain positions in the future.

Respecting rights and freedoms

Everybody in the community has rights and freedoms. In order to allow people to have their rights and freedom, we must all behave according to accepted standards of behaviour. Some of the rights of individuals and the standards of behaviour that relate to those rights are shown in the following table.

The rights of individuals	Required standards of behaviour
People's money or personal property should not be stolen. People's property should be respected.	People should be honest, fair and trustworthy, and respect each other.
People should feel safe in the community.	People should respect each other and not fight or be violent and damage property.
Disagreements will be solved in ways that are fair and reasonable to all.	People should listen to each other and be patient, tolerant and prepared to compromise.
People live in a community that has good laws, which are respected by the people and carried out by the police and courts.	Police officers, magistrates and judges should be honest, trustworthy and do their work efficiently.
The community will be served by government workers and politicians—the job they are paid or elected to do.	Public servants and politicians should not use bribery or be involved in corruption. They should not be greedy, dishonest or help themselves.
People should be able to choose good leaders and change their leaders when needed.	Leaders and electoral officers should be honest, trustworthy and carry out their work properly.
People should be able to move freely from place to place when they want.	People should not harass or attack each other. Laws should allow freedom of movement.
People should be free to follow their own religion or other beliefs.	People should be tolerant and not try to force their ideas on other people.
Children have the right to receive at least a basic education.	The government should provide schools, trained teachers and learning materials. Parents and the community should be interested in and support children's education. People will respect and care for teachers and schools.
The community has the right to health services.	The government will provide aid posts, health centres and hospitals, trained health workers and the drugs and equipment they need. People will respect and care for health workers and facilities.

The Rights of the Child

The Convention on the Rights of the Child was adopted and agreed by the General Assembly of the United Nations on 20 November 1989. It entered into force on 2 September 1990. The following list includes the articles most relevant to Papua New Guinea, expressed in simple words that children can understand:

Article 1: Everyone under the age of 18 has all the rights of this convention.

Article 2: You have these rights whoever you are, whoever your parents are, whatever colour you are, whatever sex or religion you are, whatever language you speak, whether you have a disability, or if you are rich or poor.

Article 3: Whenever an adult has anything to do with you, he or she should do what is in your best interest.

Article 6: Everyone should recognise that you have a right to live.

Article 7: You have the right to have a name, and when you are born, your name, your parents' names and the date should be written down. You have the right to a nationality and the right to know that you will be cared for by your parents.

Article 9: You should not be separated from your parents, unless it is for your own good. For instance, your parents may be hurting you or not taking care of you. Also, if your parents decide to live apart, you will have to live with one or the other of them, but you have the right to contact both parents easily.

Article 10: If you and your parents are living in separate countries, you have the right to get back together and live in the same place.

Article 11: You should not be kidnapped, and if you are, the government should try its hardest to get you back.

Article 12: Whenever adults make a decision that will affect you in any way, you have the right to give your opinion, and the adults have to take you seriously.

Article 13: You have the right to find out things and say what you think through speaking, writing, making art and so on, unless it breaks the rights of others.

Article 14: You have the right to think what you like and be whatever religion you want to be. Your parents should help you to learn what is right and wrong.

Article 15: You have the right to meet, make friends with, and make clubs with other people, unless it breaks the rights of others.

Article 16: You have the right to a private life. For instance, you can keep a diary that other people are not allowed to see.

Article 17: You have the right to collect information from radios, newspapers, television, books and so on from all around the world. Adults should make sure that you get information that you understand.

Article 18: Both your parents should be involved in bringing you up and they should do what is best for you.

Article 19: No one should hurt you in any way. Adults should make sure that you are protected from abuse, violence and neglect. Even your parents have no right to hurt you.

Article 20: If you do not have parents, or if is not safe for you to live with your parents, you have the right to special protection and help.

Article 21: If you have been adopted, adults should make sure that everything is arranged so that it is best for you.

Article 22: If you are a refugee (meaning you have to leave your own country because it is not safe for you to live there), you have the right to special protection and help.

Article 23: If you are disabled, either mentally or physically, you have the right to special care and education to help you to grow up in the same way as other children.

Article 24: You have the right to good health. This means that you should have professional care and medicines when you are sick. Adults should try their hardest to make sure that children do not get sick in the first place by feeding and taking good care of them.

Article 27: You have the right to a good enough 'standard of living'. This means that parents have the responsibility to make sure that you have food, clothes, a place to live and so on. If parents cannot afford this, the government should help.

Article 28: You have the right to education. Primary education must be free and you must go to primary school. You should also be able to go to secondary school.

Article 29: The purpose of education is to develop your personality, talents, and mental and physical abilities to the fullest. Education should also prepare you to live responsibly and peacefully, in a free society, understanding the rights of other people and respecting the environment.

Article 30: If you come from a minority group, you have the right to enjoy your own culture, practise your own religion and use your own language.

Article 31: You have the right to play.

Article 32: You have the right to be protected from working in places or conditions that are likely to damage your health or get in the way of your education. If someone is making money out of your work, you should get paid fairly.

Article 33: You have the right to be protected from illegal drugs and from the business of making and selling drugs.

Article 34: You have the right to be protected from sexual abuse. This means that nobody can do anything to your body that you do not want them to do, such as touching you or taking pictures of you or making you say things that you don't want to say.

Article 35: No one is allowed to kidnap or sell you.

Article 37: Even if you do something that is wrong, no one is allowed to punish you in a way that humiliates you or hurts you badly. You should never be put in prison except as a last resort; and if you are put in prison, you have the right to special care and regular visits from your family.

Article 38: You have the right to protection in times of war. If you are under fifteen, you should never have to be in an army or take part in a battle.

Article 39: If you have been hurt or neglected in any way—for instance, in a war—you have the right to special care and treatment.

Article 40: You have the right to defend yourself if you have been accused of committing a crime. The police, lawyers and judges in court should treat you with respect and make sure that you understand everything that is going on.

Article 42: All adults and children should know about the Convention of the Rights of the Child. You have a right to learn about rights and adults should know about them too.

What you can do

The famous anthropologist Margaret Mead once said, 'Never doubt that a small group of committed people can change the world; indeed it is the only thing that ever has.'

People who know their rights are better able to claim them. Promoting the Convention on the Rights of the Child and making its provisions widely known are therefore essential steps to realise children's rights. You or your school can help raise awareness in your community of the Convention and its aims by:

- organising meetings and distributing materials within your community about the Convention on the Rights of the Child
- working with your local churches, schools and community groups to create grass-roots support for the Convention
- urging your local and national lawmakers to provide education and training on child rights for all those working with children—teachers, medical professionals, social workers, members of the police force and other law enforcement professionals

Teachers, social workers and other professionals working with children can raise awareness of the Convention on the Rights of the Child among the children with whom they come into contact. School is a particularly important environment for creating awareness about child rights.

Appendices

This unit of work is just one way of integrating a number of learning outcomes from different strands and sub-strands of Personal Development in Grade 8. There are many other ways in which teachers can integrate learning outcomes, including those from other subjects, to make a unit of work. Teachers need to develop units of work that meet the needs of students and the community, and also suit their own teaching style. Just as we can weave bilums from different kinds of material into different shapes and sizes for different purposes, so different units of work can be planned and implemented, each with their own special characteristics.

SAMPLE UNIT OF WORK

Growing up, making friends and staying healthy

Grade: 8

Time: One term

Strand: Health of Individuals and Population

Sub-strands:

Identify and describe behaviour that promotes growth and development, taking into account heredity and environment (8.4.1).

Outline issues arising from differences in rates of growth and development and how individuals manage the changes (8.4.2).

Identify different cultural beliefs about sexuality (8.4.3).

Describe ways in which relationships form, develop, adapt and end (8.1.5).

Outline health issues that are of concern to young people (8.4.6).

Discuss safe sexual behaviours and sexual responsibilities (8.4.7).

Describe how people and facilities influence the choice of recreation, sporting and leisure activities (8.2.5).

Purpose: The purpose of this unit is to develop in young people the knowledge, skills and attitudes needed to pass through adolescence, come to terms with their sexuality, begin to form relationships and stay healthy.

Process skills	Student activities	Assessment	Number of lessons and estimated time
Gathering information	• List physical features that we get from our parents. • Describe behaviour that helps us to grow and develop. • Discuss the influence of the environment on our inherited characteristics, including the effect of parental behaviour on the baby in the uterus. • Describe the roles and responsibilities of parents. • Discuss issues arising in adolescence and how individuals cope with changes. • Discuss what is the right time to have a sexual relationship. • List the things to consider before starting a sexual relationship. • List the characteristics of a good relationship. • List health concerns of young people. • Compare the participation of girls and boys in recreational activities. Survey local community groups to identify their leisure and recreation needs.	**Assessment task** List physical features and personality characteristics that are similar to those of your mother or father. List the characteristics of a good relationship. List the health concerns of young people. **Assessment criteria** The student correctly lists characteristics inherited from parents. The student correctly lists examples of equality and examples of inequality in relationships (refer to *Personal Development Book 2*, p. 75). The student correctly identifies health concerns that relate to adolescence from a list that applies to all ages, including children and old people.	15 x 40-minute lessons for activities 5 x 30-minute lessons for assessment
Analysing information	• List different behaviours or conditions that will have a positive or negative effect on our growth and development. • Describe how our families and cultural groups influence our growth and development. • Discuss and identify ways to adjust to changes in relationships. • Identify positive strategies in solving health problems and making decisions. • Discuss how other people can influence an individual and their sexual behaviour. • Discuss how HIV/AIDS can influence others and how it affects lives in the community. • Discuss how to encourage girls to participate more in physical activities. • Compare different community requirements for participation in recreational and leisure activities.	**Assessment task** List and classify issues concerning adolescence. Classify a list of community requirements for participation in recreational and leisure activities. **Assessment criteria** The student correctly lists and classifies issues common in adolescence. The student correctly classifies community requirements for participation in recreational and leisure activities according to physical (facilities and equipment), economic (affordability) and social/cultural (gender, age, disability etc.) requirements.	15 x 40-minute lessons for activities 5 x 30-minute lessons for assessment

Process skills	Student activities	Assessment	Number of lessons and estimated time
Action taken	• Make personal decisions and take action on issues related to personal growth and development. • Use the decision-making model that you learned in Living and Working in Grade 6 to discuss with a partner what you would do to sort out different problems or issues. • Practise skills needed for handling the changes that occur during adolescence. • Write down strategies to cope with pressure to have a sexual relationship. • Describe strategies to deal with ending a relationship, such as that with a boyfriend of girlfriend. • Discuss ways to prevent STIs and HIV/AIDS.	**Assessment task** Match specific skills that are needed to handle the changes that affect adolescents. Describe ways to prevent STIs, HIV/AIDS. **Assessment criteria** Student correctly matches a list of skills needed with changes that occur during adolescence. Student correctly identifies behaviour that will prevent the spread of STIs, including HIV/AIDS, from a list of behaviours.	15 x 40-minute lessons for activities 4 x 30-minute lessons for assessment

Resources: *National Curriculum Statement, Personal Development Upper Primary Syllabus 2003, Personal Development Upper Primary Teachers Guide 2003, Personal Development Teacher Resource, Personal Development Book 2.*

Suggested links with other subjects or strands within Personal Development: Health of Individuals and Population; Relationships; Our Culture, Lifestyle and Values.

Total estimated time for the unit of work: 45 x 40-minute teaching periods; 14 x 30-minute periods for assessment. (Total: 2220 minutes: i.e., approximately the equivalent of one term's work for Personal Development.)

Planning templates

Following are some sample templates that can be used in both long- and short-term planning.

Sample 1: Yearly plan

Strand	Term 1	Term 2	Term 3	Term 4
Relationships	Changing roles and responsibilities	Interactions in relationships and groups	Cultural and personal identity	Managing relationships
Movement and Physical Activity	Roles and responsibilities	Leisure and recreation	Safety and movement skills	Fitness for health
Our Culture, Lifestyle and Values	Culture and values	Culture and values	Lifestyle and changes	Lifestyle and changes
Health of Individuals and Population	Growth and development	Personal health and safety	Nutrition Use of drugs	Community health
Living and Working Together	Respecting rights and freedoms	Making choices	Rule of law	Good and fair leaders

Sample 2: Term plan

Week	Student tasks	Required resources	Assessment procedures
1–3			
4–6			
7–10			

Sample 3: Lesson plan

Teaching group Individual Whole class Team group √	**Required materials**
Learning strategies Collaborating Interpreting Predicting Planning √ Investigating Recording √ Justifying Changing Communicating √	**Specific content—lesson plan**
Learning outcomes	**Assessment tasks**
Related outcomes from other subjects	**Integrated activities**

Defining terms

Assessment refers to the collection and analysis of data about student behaviour and progress. Assessment data can also be used to make program decisions.

Evaluation refers to the process of using assessment information to make judgments about the effectiveness of teaching programs and to improve teaching practice so as to improve student learning.

Reporting refers to the procedures whereby assessment information is communicated to others (usually parents, students and other teachers) to inform and assist student learning.

Record-keeping is the documentation we keep when we assess and evaluate. Assessment information needs to be recorded in ways which enable the teacher to construct a profile of learning for each child.

An **Outcome** can be defined as a behaviour that students will demonstrate after learning experiences. Outcomes generally relate to knowledge and skills. Outcomes are usually broad and relate to long-term learning. Outcomes are demonstrable, sequential and observable.

Assessment templates

The following templates are designed to give teachers suggestions on recording assessment information. They are not meant to be prescriptive, but to assist teachers in designing their own assessment records.

Sample 1: Skills assessment template

PERSONAL DEVELOPMENT—SKILLS CHECKLIST

NAME: **DATE:**

Topic	Skills	Achieved √			Comments
		Most of the time	Some of the time	Rarely	
Relationships	research and gather information conduct surveys use questionnaires analyse information evaluate results analyse different groups and their influence communicate and cooperate with others develop skills to make good decisions negotiate and handle family and group issues in positive and peaceful ways express feelings use assertive, non-aggressive communication resolve conflict demonstrate positive attitudes and skills clarify own values think critically describe different roles and responsibilities role play demonstrate cooperative and sharing skills evaluate issues and act appropriately				
Movement and Physical Activity	(Insert your own list of skills here)				
Our Culture, Lifestyle and Values	(Insert your own list of skills here)				
Health of Individuals and Populations	(Insert your own list of skills here)				
Living and Working	(Insert your own list of skills here)				

Sample 2: Cognitive skills template

LEARNING SKILLS ASSESSMENT CHECKLIST

For assessing learning skills, group communication skills and attitudes

NAME: **DATE:**

Skills	Skills observed √	Comments
Learning skills • can form and ask questions • can follow instructions • can find information • can find required information • can express ideas clearly and correctly • can critically reflect on own work • can organise self efficiently • understands how to improve own work • manages use of time well		
Group skills • follows group rules • works cooperatively within a team • contributes to discussions without dominating • listens while other people speak • accommodates different points of view		
Attitudes • respects other students' point of view • participates freely in activities • works in a constructive and positive way • values the beliefs held by other students		

Sample 3: Student self-assessment template

STUDENT SELF-ASSESSMENT CHECKLIST

NAME: **DATE:**

Skills	Can do √
My learning skills • I can ask questions • I can follow instructions • I can find the information that I need • I can express myself clearly and correctly • I can think about what was right and wrong about my work • I can work neatly • I am well organised • I understand how to improve my work • I use my time well	
My group skills • I can work well with others in a group • I can listen when others are talking • I can discuss something without getting angry	
My attitude • I can listen and respect what others have to say • I can take responsibility for my own work • I can share in a group activity • I can learn from my mistakes	

My comments

Sample 4: Group assessment template

GROUP ASSESSMENT TEMPLATE

Date: ____

Names of group members:

____

____

____

Name of group: ________________________________

Activity:

____

____

____

What things did your group do really well?

____

____

____

What things does your group need to do to improve?

____

____

____

What are you going to do to change the way your group works?

____

____

Sample 5: Term self-assessment template

MY TERM REPORT

NAME:

I rate my working habits this term as:

I am a quiet worker	/10
I am a neat worker	/10
I finish my work on time	/10
I am able to work by myself	/10
I work well in groups	/10

What I did well this term

What I plan to improve on next term

What I would like to see changed next term

What I really liked doing this term

What I didn't like doing this term

Additional Projects and Investigations

Relationships (Year 6)

1 Find out more about village constables, luluais and tultuls. When did Papua New Guinea have these? What did they do? Why do we not have them today? Make a poster about luluais and tultuls, with pictures, and display it in your classroom.

2 Ask old people in your community about the times of the village constables, luluais and tultuls.

3 Invite an older person to come to the school to talk to the students about what life was like in previous times. What did people do? How did people live? How were things different then?
If possible, ask them to show you some of things that people used years ago in their homes or in their work, or to show you some old pictures or old papers. Remember that we need to be careful with old things because they can sometimes be easily broken.

4 Find out about Cooperative Societies in your area. If there are any old people who have been members of Cooperative Societies invite them to come and talk to your class.

How did members of the Cooperative Society help each other? What do you think happened to Cooperative Societies? Why do we not see Cooperative Societies in Papua New Guinea today?

5 Put the following in increasing size, from the group with the smallest number of members to the group with the largest number.

clan village nation province family tribe

6 Do you agree or disagree with the following statements? Give reasons for your answer.

a All people can be placed into groups

b We use similarities and differences to put people into groups

c People can belong to more than one group

d We can always choose which groups we belong to

e Achievements are not important.

7 a Classify the words below into those groups of which we have a choice to be a member, and those groups of which we do not have a choice to be a member.

small	clown	son	granddaughter	groups
achievements	cousins	daughter	classmates	best friend

b From the same list find the words that are missing from the passage below:

Everybody belongs to different ____________________. For example, if you are a boy then you must also be a ____________________ to your parents, or if you are a girl you must also be a ____________________. As your grandparents get old they may start to forget some things, but they will never forget that you are their grandson or ____________________. If you live near your uncles and aunts then you will probably enjoy playing with your ____________________. When you go to school all the other children in your class will be your ____________________. Some of these may be taller than you and others may be ____________________. In many classes there is a boy or girl who makes the other students laugh a lot and he or she is often known as a

_________________. Many boys and girls have a ______________________ at school – someone that they really like and play with a lot. Students who get good marks at school and are good at sport are often recognised for their ______________________.

8 Make a table like the one below and list the roles and responsibilities of the people in your school. You can include the teachers and anyone else who comes into the school to help, like parents.

Person	Roles and responsibilities
Head teacher	
Deputy	
Class teacher	
Class captain	
Sports captain	
Student	

9 Classify the following behaviours into those that help to solve problems and that do not help to solve problems.

- Fighting
- Running away
- Admitting that you were wrong
- Telling lies
- Saying that you are sorry
- Trying to discuss sensibly
- Giving in easily
- Blaming somebody else
- Inviting someone to take part in something you know they will like
- Keeping quiet and refusing to talk
- Asking someone who is not involved to help sort out the problem
- Sulking
- Sharing food or a drink with the other person
- Pretending to be really angry when you are not
- Breaking things
- Keeping calm and trying to think carefully
- Ignoring the problem or pretending that nothing is happening
- Telling stories behind the back of the other person

Relationships (Years 7 and 8)

1 Write down the family tree for your family or work out the family tree for a well-known family.

2 Find out more about different kinds of families in other countries.

3 Invite an older person to come to the school to talk to the students about family life in previous times. What was the place of children and grandparents? How did people choose a husband or wife? How were things different then?

If possible, ask them to show you some of things that people used years ago in their homes or in their work, or to show you some old pictures or old papers. Remember that we need to be careful with old things because they can sometimes easily be broken.

4 Find out about equality in Papua New Guinea in places where men and women work. When they do the same work, do they earn the same money? Talk to people who are working or to employers, or find out from job advertisements in newspapers.

5 Invite someone from your community who is a role model to come and give a talk at your school. Ask them how they came to be in their position. Did they have role models? In their behaviour, are they always aware that other people may be watching them?

6 Carry out a survey in your community to find out what standards of behaviour are important.

7 Carry out a survey in your community to find out what people think are the characteristics of a good friendship.

8 Social indicators help to tell us about equality and inequality in a community. We can use social indicators to compare communities and populations. Six social indicators for six countries are shown in the graphs of the *Personal Development Student Book 2* on page 172. For each graph, describe the position of Papua New Guinea for that social indicator in relation to the other countries.

9 Using the words in the list, find the words that are missing from the passage below. You can use each word only once.

skills countries family families different similarities role

We are all members of a family although there are many different types of ____________________. Families can be ____________________ in the same country and can also be different in other ____________________ in the world. People play different roles in each ____________________ and there is an accepted code of behaviour for each relationship and group. People can be described by their ____________________ to and differences from each other. People take on different roles in a family. When we take on a particular ____________________, this affects our relationships, attitude and behaviour. Relationships are important in families and ____________________ are needed to maintain effective relationships.

Movement and physical activity (Year 6)

1 Carry out a survey to find out about sports injuries in your school or community. Use a record sheet like the one below.

Sport	What happened? (Who? Where? When?)	What care can be taken in future? How can this be prevented?

Make a summary of your findings and tell the rest of the class.

2 Help to organise some 'keeping fit' activities for particular groups in the community.

3 Plan and carry out a mini-sports competition for children in your community. Do this to help celebrate an important day like Independence Anniversary, your provincial day or Christmas Day.

4 Learn and perform some traditional dancing to celebrate an important day like Independence Anniversary, your provincial day or the end of the school year. You will need to plan and practice for some weeks before the event. People from the local community could be invited to teach the dances and to take part in the celebration.

5 Using the words in the list, find the words that are missing from the passage below. You can use each word only once.

exercise	injured fit	fair	fun	
fitness	movement	recreation	roles	abilities

When we take part in games, sports and dance we need to learn a range of ________________ skills. When we learn sequences of movements we need to think about the different ____________________ that people have. Being ____________________ means being able to take part in everyday activities without getting tired. ____________________ and eating the right kind of food help people to be fit. Rules and safety procedures in games and sport help to prevent people being ____________________ and make the game ____________________. Leisure and ____________________ are activities that people do on their own or in groups to have ____________________ and relax, to make new friends, or to develop ______________. In some games and in organised sport, people have different ____________________ and responsibilities.

6 Which of the following skills are important in netball and basketball?

A. Throwing the ball

B. Catching the ball

C. Throwing and catching

D. Dribbling and fielding

7 Floating and sculling in water are important because

A. They help to win swimming races

B. They help to prevent drowning

C. They help people to get good exercise

D. They give good rhythm and coordination

8 In which of the following sports is dribbling an important skill?

A. Netball and softball

B. Cricket and volleyball

C. Rugby and swimming

D. Soccer and basketball

9 Which of the following are skills that are common to both dancing and sport?

A. Rhythm and timing

B. Dribbling and passing

C. Combining movements in a sequence

D. Making decisions quickly

(a) A only

(b) D only

(c) A and B

(d) A and C

10 Which of the following best describes the sequence of skills that you would use in doing the long jump?

A. Do not put your foot over the line
B. Land on your feet and do not touch the sand with any part of your body
C. Run fast toward the take-off point
D. Keep moving forward away from the pit
(a) A, B, C, D
(b) B, A, C, D
(c) C, A, B, D
(d) C, B, A, D

11 What does it mean to be fit?

A. Taking part in activities without feeling tired
B. Getting your breath back quickly after exercise
C. Relaxing your mind and muscles
D. Feeling happy and energetic
E. Getting along well with others
(a) A and B only
(b) A, B, C and D only
(c) B, C, D and E only
(d) A, B, C, D and E

12 Which of the following activities help to promote fitness?

A. Working in the garden and walking
B. Eating the right kind of food and having a good diet
C. Chewing betel nut and smoking tobacco
D. Getting enough sleep and rest
(a) A, B and C only
(b) A, B and D only
(c) A, C and D only
(d) A, B, C and D

13 What is the purpose of rules and safety procedures in sport?

A. To make the game fair for the players
B. To make the game safe for the players
C. To make the game safe for the spectators
D. To make sure that there is a clear winner
(a) A and B only
(b) C and D only
(c) A, B and C only
d) A, B, C and D

14 Copy and complete the following table. Which of the following are the responsibilities of team members and which are the responsibility of the coach? If something is the responsibility of both player and coach then you can tick both.

Responsibility	Player	Coach
Attend training		
Perform to the best of their ability		
Help players to develop their skills and fitness		
Follow instructions		
Turn up for practices and games on time		
Discipline players – tell them when they are doing right or wrong		
Support other players or performers		
Ensure a safe environment to prevent injury		
Report things that may cause danger, accidents or other problems		
Encourage fair play		

Movement and Physical Activity (Years 7 and 8)

1 Organise a novelty sports day at your school to celebrate the end of term or a special day. Possible events are:
   - Egg and spoon race—you can use any round object like betel nuts instead of eggs. (If you have a plastic spoon, try carrying it in your mouth instead of your hand.)
   - Sack race—use copra sacks or coffee sacks
   - Wheelbarrow race—one person 'walks' along on her hands while her legs are supported by her partner
   - Three-legged race—two people tie two of their legs together with a strip of cloth
   - Carrying balloons filled with water between the knees
   - Hoopla—throw wire rings over a tin or bottle.
   - Throwing balls in the bucket—you can make your own balls from coconut leaves or rolling up a number of plastic shopping bags and tying them together.
   - Pushing a bar of soap up a slippery slope with a stick
   - A slow bicycle race—if you have only two bicycles you can have heats
   - Tunnel ball

2 Learn how to give first aid when it is needed. If you do not know how to give first aid, then invite someone to come to the school to teach you.

3 Ask your teacher to invite someone to come to your school to teach self-defence.

4 Carry out a survey to find out about the need for leisure and recreation activities in your school or community. Use a record sheet like the one below.

Leisure activity or recreation	How could this be organised? (Who? Where? When?)	What is needed to make this activity happen?

Make a summary of your findings and tell the rest of the class.

5 Help to organise some 'keeping fit' activities for particular groups in the community.

6 Plan and carry out a mini-sports competition for children in your community. Do this to help celebrate an important day like Independence Anniversary, your provincial day or Christmas Day.

7 Learn and perform some traditional dancing to celebrate an important day like Independence Anniversary, your provincial day or the end of the school year. You will need to plan and practise for some weeks before the event. People from the local community could be invited to teach the dances and to take part in the celebration.

8 Choose a game that is played in your area and play the game, looking for the strategies and tactics that the players use when playing the game. Develop a checklist that you can use to help make and record your observations easily after the game. What conclusions can you make from your observations?

9 Develop a personal fitness program for a number of different people. For example:

A younger brother or sister

An older brother or sister

Your parents

Elderly people

People who are very inactive

People with a disability

10 Choose a game that is played in your area and play the game, looking for the risks that the players take and the rules and safety procedures that are followed in order to reduce the risk. Develop a checklist that you can use to help make and record your observations easily after the game.
- What conclusions can you make from your observations?
- How can the game be made safer?

11 Carry out a survey of any leisure or recreation facilities in your area. Develop a simple form to find the answer to questions such as:
- Who uses the facilities?
- When are they available?
- Are the facilities safe to use?
- Is the equipment that is needed for the activity complete and in working order?
- etc.

Write up a report to summarise your findings.

12 Choose a game that is played in your area and play the game, looking for the ways that the team communicates and cooperates. Develop a checklist that you can use to help make and record your observations easily after the game. What conclusions can you make from your observations?

13 Choose a game that you and your friends like to play. Work out a system of signs or words to communicate with your team-mates about particular moves in the game so that members of the other team will not easily understand. Draw a table with symbols and a key to explain to your team-mates how the system will work.

Example: Basketball

Move 1:
- Player with the ball calls out 'eight'.
- Player with the ball passes it behind the player from the other side who then passes it back to the first player.

Example: Touch

Move 1: The acting-half pass

Watch the ball. Place both hands on the ball and gently swing it from the ground to the receiver. Signal to the team by putting the left foot forward for a pass to the right and the right foot forward for a pass to the left.

14 Using the words in the list, find the words that are missing from the passage below. You can use each word only once.

people movements different roles activities emergencies dangerous plans

To take part in games, sports and dance we need to link a range of ____________________ skills together. Skills often involve sequences of movements. When we learn sequences of ____________________, we need to develop good body control. Taking part in a variety of physical ____________________ helps to develop different parts of our fitness. Some sporting activities can be ____________________ and we need to know how to deal with dangerous situations and with ____________________. People are sometimes slow to take part in recreational and leisure activities, and in order to encourage them to take part, suitable ____________________ are needed. Many different ____________________ can be involved in organising sports. In some games and in organised sport, there are different codes of behaviour for the various ____________________ that people take.

Our culture, lifestyle and values (Year 6)

1 Find out more about the Hiri or the Kula Ring. Which groups of people were involved? What was exchanged? Why were these trading voyages important to the people who took part in them? Do they still take place today?

- Invite someone from Central Province or Milne Bay to come and talk about traditional trade.
- Find out about the Hiri Moale festival in Port Moresby.

2 Find out about the Moka pig-killing ceremony in the Southern Highlands. Write a short story to answer the following: What happens? Who is involved? Why is it important?

3 Invite elders from the community to come and talk about the changes that they have noticed. Which changes do they feel happy about and which changes do they feel unhappy about?

What can people do about the changes that are not good changes?

4 Using the words in the list, find the words that are missing from the passage below. You can use each word only once.

subsistence	gardens	exchanging	country	barter
culture	changes	languages	traditional	trading

In Papua New Guinea, the ____________________ of the people is still strong and there are many differences in the culture of people from different parts of the ____________________. There are many different kinds of people with different ____________________, cultures and traditions. In many places, people are still living a ____________________ way of life, but there are also many ____________________ taking place. For example, people who grow food in their ____________________, go fishing and hunting, make their own clothing and build houses from bush materials are sometimes called ____________________. When people from different places first moved about, one of the ways that they came to know each other was through ____________________. Trading means ____________________ something you have for something that someone else has, and which you want. When people trade or swap one type of goods for another type of goods, the exchange is sometimes called ____________________.

Our Culture, Lifestyle and Values (Years 7 and 8)

1 Visit a site near your school where there have been many changes. Identify and list the changes. Which changes are positive and which are negative?

2 Invite elders from the community to come and talk about the changes that they have noticed in the environment. Which changes do they feel happy about and which changes do they feel unhappy about? What can people do about the changes that are not good changes?

3 Find out about the physical, social and economic changes that have taken place in other places and note the causes for those changes.

4 Choose your own community or a community that you know well. Work out a time line to show the customs associated with the seasons, with planting and harvesting of food crops or with other important occasions in the community such as weddings and funerals.

5 Write a letter to invite elders from the community to come and talk about the way that the lifestyle of the people in the area has changed. Show the letter to your teacher before you send it.

6 Invite someone who has lived overseas to come and talk about the way of life of the people in the place where they lived.

7 Invite visitors or people from other places to come and visit your school and talk about their lifestyle. For example, if you live in a place where there are tourists or people travelling on a yacht, you could invite them to come and talk to the students in your school.

8 Using the words in the list, find the words that are missing from the passage below. You can use each word only once.

changes different country life traditions forgotten

Customs, rituals and ____________________ are still strong in Papua New Guinea, but some may be lost or ____________________. There are many differences in the culture of people from ____________________ parts of the country. We should respect our own culture and that of people from other parts of the ____________________ and from other countries. As Papua New Guinea develops, many ____________________ are taking place to the way of ____________________ of people, and some of these are affecting the culture.

9 Answer true or false to the following statements about changes that are happening to our way of life.

a Roads allow people to move about more easily, to buy and sell goods and to reach schools and hospitals.

b New food crops and farming methods decrease the variety of food available.

c New cash crops allow people to earn money.

d Electricity for lights and cooking is important to help keep people healthy.

e A reliable water supply makes life easier and helps to keep people healthy.

f Closing of Aid Posts can affect the health of the community.

g Clearing land for logging or mining can cause damage to land, rivers and wildlife, and loss of farming land.

Health of Individuals and Population (Year 6)

1 If your school has a tuck shop or canteen, carry out a survey to find out whether it sells good snack foods or 'rubbish' foods. If it sells 'rubbish' foods make some suggestions about other, more healthy foods that could be sold.

If there is no tuck shop or canteen in your school, carry out a survey to find out if there is a need for one.

2 In your class or your school, plan and carry out a long-term project to improve the health of the school or community. For example:

- install or repair water tanks
- install or repair guttering to collect rainwater
- repair taps – for example, replace washers
- build new or better toilets
- organise better rubbish disposal
- make better drains

Parents and citizens could get involved in such a project.

3 Choose a health problem in your school or in the community. Plan some simple activities that can be used to help people to behave in ways that are more healthy. Show your plans to the other students and your teacher. Choose the best ideas and put them into practice.

4 Some schools have become Health Promoting Schools. What do we mean by Health Promoting Schools? Is your school a Health Promoting School? Invite someone to come and talk about Health Promoting Schools.

5 Invite a good role model to come to your school and talk about why he or she does not take harmful drugs. This could be a person who has never taken harmful drugs or someone who took harmful drugs in the past but no longer takes them.

6 Using the words in the list, find the words that are missing from the passage below. You can use each word only once.

washing	surroundings	adolescence	immunisations	development	balanced
adulthood	characteristics	infancy	drugs germs	treat	dangers

We all pass through key stages in our ____________________: from birth, through ____________________ and childhood, into puberty and ____________________, then into ____________________ and old age, and finally death. We all get ____________________ from our parents, but we are also affected by our ____________________ as we grow up. Eating healthy food and a ____________________ diet, taking regular exercise and getting enough rest will help us to grow properly and stay healthy. ____________________ ourselves and our clothes, sheets and towels regularly, and keeping our surroundings clean also help us to stay healthy. Illnesses can be spread by ____________________ and we can prevent sickness by keeping clean, having vaccinations or ____________________ and getting treatment when we are sick. There are ____________________ at school and at home, and we need to learn how to avoid these and stay safe. Drugs or medicines can help to prevent sickness and can be used to ____________________ people who are sick. Some ____________________, like betel nut, tobacco and alcohol, can make people sick.

7 List two advantages and two disadvantages of each of the places that you can get information about sexual development in the table below.

Places that you get information about sexual development	Advantages	Disadvantages
books		
friends and peers		
teachers		
parents and elders		
newspapers, magazines, radio, television, video		

8 In the table below, classify each food according to the group to which it belongs (some may belong to more than one group).

Food/drink	Energy food	Body-building food (protein)	Protective food
taro			
fish			
coconut milk			
white rice			
chicken			
beans			
pawpaw			
sago			
aibika			
corned beef			
mango			
peanuts			
corn			
pork			
eggs			
milk			
margarine			
tomato			

Health of Individuals and Population (Years 7 and 8)

1 Write down a question about growth and development on a piece of paper. Do not put your name on the paper. Put the paper in a box. Later on your teacher will go through the questions and sort them out. Your teacher will read out each question and talk about the answers with the class.

2 Invite a guest speaker from the community to talk about local customs and rules related to food.

3 Make a plan for the sale of healthy food on special occasions like Independence Anniversary and end of year celebrations. Carry out your plan.

4 In your class or your school, plan and carry out a long-term project to improve the environment of the school or community. For example:
- Plant fruit trees around the school or community.
- Plant shade trees around the school or community.
- Start a nursery for fruit trees and shade trees.
- Build better toilets.
- Organise better rubbish disposal.
- Construct better drains.

Parents and citizens could get involved in such a project.

5 Choose a health problem in your school or in the community. Plan some simple activities that can be used to help people to behave in ways that are more healthy. Show your plans to the other students

and your teacher. Choose the best ideas and put them into practice.

6 Invite someone from the Health Department to come and talk about the health problems and social problems that can happen when people take drugs.

7 If students in your class have missed out on vaccinations, your teacher may organise a visit to the local health centre or hospital.

8 Plan and cook a nutritious meal for a special occasion and invite some parents from the community to come and share the meal. Or invite some mothers from the community to cook a nutritious meal for your class.

9 Plan a nutrition day for your school. Advertise the day by making posters to put up in the community or by making announcements. Activities could include displays of different kinds of foods, cooking demonstrations, nutritious food to buy and eat, recipes, and stories or poems about food.

10 Invite someone from the local health centre or from the local community to come and give a demonstration on how to plan and prepare nutritious meals using only foods that are available in the local area.

11 Think about the way that people live in your community. Plan and carry out a program to help people to follow healthy practices and live more safely in the community.

12 Invite an older person from the community to come and discuss family life in the past and compare it with the present. How many children were in a family then? How was life different?

13 Look at the maps of PNG on pages 176–7 of the *Personal Development Student Book 2* which give information about four health issues in 1994.
- From the information given, which provinces have the best health services? Give reasons for your choice.
- From the information given, which provinces are likely to have the greatest health problems? Give reasons for your choice.

14 Look at the graphs showing cases of diseases preventable by immunisation (1990–93) and total vaccinations (1990–94).
- From the graphs, what are the most important preventable diseases?
- From the graphs, which vaccination program reaches the most children?
- For measles, compare the total vaccinations given with the cases of the disease. What conclusions can you make?

15 Using the words in the list, find the words that are missing from the passages below. You can use each word only once.

illness	appearance	plan	alcohol	community	behave	choices
negative	reproductive	food	drugs	effect		

The main purpose of the ____________________ system is to allow men and women to have children. When we grow up from girls into women and from boys into men, many changes take place in our ____________________ and in the way that we feel and behave. The way that we ____________________ can increase or reduce the respect that we have for each other.

Eating is a behaviour that varies in people from different places. People eat different kinds of ____________________ and eat in different ways. Everyone can ____________________ healthy and nutritious meals using food that is available locally.

We can make plans and ____________________ about our own health using our knowledge about what makes us sick. We can keep ourselves healthy by avoiding ____________________ and other risky situations that threaten our personal health and safety. Our behaviour should not have a negative effect on the health of other people in the ____________________. We can also help others in the community to learn about health and safety and to prevent ____________________.

Because of the ways that we live, we are having an effect on the environment, which in turn is having an ____________________ on our health. Drugs can also affect the health of people who use them and have a ____________________ effect on other people in the community. Each person has a choice about whether he or she will use drugs and ____________________.

16 Answer true or false to the following statements.

a The stage in life when you develop into an adult is called puberty.

b Adolescence begins before puberty.

c Puberty usually begins in boys about two years before girls.

d Having periods is a normal thing that happens to every girl.

e When boys and girls grow up, they become taller and heavier and hair begins to grow under the arm and in the pubic area.

f When a boy starts to produce sperm, it is possible for him to become a father.

g When a girl starts to have periods, it is possible for her to become a mother.

17 In the following list, put a tick in the appropriate column to show which behaviour encourages respect and which reduces respect.

Behaviour	Encourages respect	Reduces respect
Shouting or using bad language		
Greeting someone by smiling and shaking hands		
Interrupting other people and not letting them give their point of view		
Being humble and not putting yourself above other people		
Calling people names		
Putting other people first by helping them		
Being aggressive and wanting to fight		
Refusing to talk about important issues		
Comforting or caring for people who are sick or old		
Agreeing to do something and then not doing it		
Listening to different points of view		
Being selfish and trying to get the best for yourself		
Accepting that there can be more than one correct answer or more than one way of doing something—not just your way		

18 Answer true or false to the following statements.

a Children who are still growing need to eat plenty of protein food.

b Women who are pregnant need to eat less protein and foods like milk that contain calcium, which can harm the baby.

c People who are very active, do hard physical work or play sport need to eat more energy food.

d People who are sick need to eat more food to help them get better.

e People living in a hot place need to eat more energy food than people living in a cold place.

f People living in hot places need to drink plenty of liquids.

19 Which of the following are ways to protect yourself and others from harm and stay healthy? Answer true or false.

a Smoke cigarettes with your friends because you want to feel part of the group.

b When you are old enough to drink alcohol, drink only a little.

c Ignore the warning on the bottle about drinking methylated spirits.

d Say 'no' to drugs like marijuana.

e Keep dangerous objects and substances like kerosene and medicines away from children.

f Follow the rules when doing any activity that can be dangerous.

g Go to places where it is unsafe.

h Follow instructions on medicines and bottles of cleaning materials, and other signs.

i Follow directions and given by people in authority like parents, teachers and the police.

Living and working together (Year 6)

1 Invite a councillor or other respected person from the community to come and talk about the value of different rules and laws.

2 Invite a policeman or policewoman to come and talk about their work in the community.

3 If your school is near a town, find out when the District Court or National Court is sitting and arrange a visit to the court. Or invite a magistrate to visit your school and talk about the work of the courts.

4 Use a questionnaire like the one below to carry out a survey about the attitudes of students in your school and people in the local community. Some questions have been included, but you can write more of your own.

Question	Strongly agree	Agree	Disagree	Strongly disagree
People who break the law should be punished				
Everyone is free to do as they please				
People should feel safe everywhere they go				
Girls do not have the same freedom as boys				
Rules should be different for boys and girls				
The biggest problem in the community is people breaking the law				

5 Using the words in the list, find the words that are missing from the passage below. You can use each word only once.

behaviour community leader freedoms useful influences

rights qualities laws decisions

People have different ____________________. These qualities can help them to be a good and ____________________ member of a group. Not everybody can be a leader, and to be a good and fair ____________________ the person must have certain qualities. Everybody must follow the rules and laws of the ____________________. These rules and laws guide our ____________________. Rules and ____________________ help to protect us and keep us safe. All people also have ____________________ and freedoms, and we must also respect the rights and ____________________ of other people. Everybody can make good ____________________ in their life by following certain steps. There are different ____________________ on the way that we make decisions.

6 In the right hand column, write down words that are the opposite of the positive qualities of a group member shown in the left hand column.

Positive quality of a group member	Negative quality of a group member
Fair	
Loyal or faithful	
Helpful	
Hard working	
Kind	
Caring	
Trustworthy	
Honest	
Reliable	

Living and Working Together (Years 7 and 8)

1 If there is a service organisation nearby, like a Rotary Club or Apex Club, invite someone to come to the school to talk about his or her community service in the area.

2 Invite someone from the community to come and talk about the value of different rules and laws.

3 Invite a policeman or policewoman to come and talk about his or her work in the community.

4 If your school is near a town, find out when the District Court or National Court is sitting and arrange a visit to the court. Or invite a magistrate to visit your school and talk about the work of the courts.

5 Use a questionnaire like the one below to carry out a survey about the attitudes of students in your school and people in the local community. Some questions have been included but you can write more of your own.

	Strongly agree	Agree	Disagree	Strongly disagree
All of the laws in PNG are good laws				
There should be different laws for different people				
Too many leaders in PNG do not follow the Leadership Code				
Leaders who break the law should be punished				

6 Invite a provincial or national politician to come to your school and talk about the way that politicians are elected. You could invite someone who has held a position in the past or someone who is currently holding a position.

7 Find out more about welfare services that are available in other countries. Why are there few welfare services in Papua New Guinea? What can we do to help provide these services?

8 Choose some different groups in Papua New Guinea and find out more about their rights.

9 Using the words in the list, find the words that are missing from the passages below. You can use each word only once.

ourselves	rights	active	positive	choose	live	freedom
community	leader	choices	roles			

When we take an ____________________ part in the community in which we live, then we help everyone else in the ____________________. There are many things that we can ____________________to do in the community in order to help others. When we make choices, there can be both ____________________ and negative results which come from those ____________________ . Some choices may affect only ____________________ and other choices will affect other people in the community.

Leaders in the community have particular ____________________ and responsibilities, and the community has expectations about the way that a ____________________ carries out his or her role. Rules and laws are needed to give people the right and ____________________ to live safely and be protected against other people. If ____________________ and freedoms are taken away, then people will be afraid and will not be able to ____________________safely together.

10 Which of the following are things that good leaders should do? Answer true or false.

- **a** Be responsible and ready to answer for the way that they behave
- **b** Help the people who are closest to them, like family and friends
- **c** Be open and honest in dealing with other people
- **d** Behave in ways to show that they are better than other people
- **e** Communicate openly with the community
- **f** Understand the needs and rights of everyone in the community
- **g** Listen to the community and to what other leaders say
- **h** Be prepared to make decisions that most people in the community do not support

Glossary

absolute majority more than half the votes which have been cast in an election.
achievement an activity which has been completed successfully.
addiction being dependent on taking drugs.
adolescence the period between puberty and maturity when children change into adults.
aggressive behaviour actions or manners that can lead to fighting.
AIDS (Acquired Immune Deficiency Syndrome) a sickness caused by the Human Immuno-deficiency Virus (HIV) that can be transmitted in semen, vaginal fluid and blood. Most people who catch HIV in Papua New Guinea catch it by having sexual intercourse with someone who has the virus. People can be infected with the virus and show no signs or symptoms for many years. There is no cure for AIDS and most people with AIDS die.
alcohol alcohol is found in beer, wines and spirits and can also be used as an antiseptic or a preservative.
alcoholic a person who has become dependent on alcohol. Because alcohol affects the brain, physical skills, memory and judgment will also be affected, which can affect relationships with other people. Drinking a lot of alcohol for many years can also affect the liver and even cause death.
anaemia a lack of red blood cells so that the blood cannot carry enough oxygen in the body.
antibiotics a kind of medicine that is made from microbes and used to cure a person who has a sickness caused by bacteria or fungi.
assertive behaviour positive behaviour in which you stand up for your rights.
attack trying to score points or goals against another team in a game of sport.
attitude our approach or thoughts and feelings about something.
bacteria small living organisms that are found in the air, in water, on food and in the ground. Some bacteria can make people sick, but sicknesses caused by bacteria can usually be cured with antibiotics. *See* antibiotics.
bagi a small red shell that is often made into necklaces.
balanced diet *See* diet.
ballot paper a paper used in an election on which a person can mark his or her vote.
balls *See* testicles.
blended family after someone dies or after a couple get divorced, a man or woman might get married again. When both husband and wife have children from the previous marriage, then they all live together. This type of family is becoming more common in developed countries.
bribery paying money or giving things to people so that they will do something for you.
candidate a person standing for election who people can vote for.
carbohydrate a type of food such as sugar and starch which provides energy in the diet.
characteristics qualities that are typical of a person or some other living thing or object.
coach someone who teaches or trains others, for example, in sport.
code of behaviour the ways that we are expected to behave with different people.
components the smaller parts of something that together make the whole.
conception the start of pregnancy when a sperm fertilises an egg in the Fallopian tube. *See* fertilisation.
concern being kind and interested in other people.
conflict the problems or disagreements that we have with other people.
constipation when people find it difficult or painful to go to the toilet, or when they have hard faeces, then we say they have constipation or are constipated.
contraception a method of preventing pregnancy.
Cooperative Society business owned and controlled by local people in Papua New Guinea.
coordination to make different things happen at the same time.
corruption *See* bribery.
customs the traditions or way of life of people.

de facto a man and woman living together, although they are not married. There may be children in this family, or the couple may not have children.

dedication being keen and loyal and willing to work hard.

defend trying to prevent the other team scoring points or goals in a game of sport.

dehydration not enough water in the body. This may be caused by sweating, vomiting or diarrhoea. The dehydrated person may not have much energy, but they do not always feel thirsty and young children can die when they are dehydrated. The treatment is to drink plenty of water with a little sugar added, but in some cases a health worker may need to put a drip in the person's arm.

dengue also called breakbone fever. A sickness caused by a virus and carried by some mosquitoes that bite in the daytime. It causes a fever and pain in the bones.

dependence (drug dependence) the effect produced when taking a drug becomes a habit. This may include alcohol and 'hard' drugs like heroin and cocaine as well as 'soft' drugs such as tobacco and marijuana.

development 1 the changes that take place in people as they grow from children into adults.
2 the changes that take place in a country.

diabetes a disease in which the person cannot use sugars properly to produce energy. Sugar appears in the urine and the person is thirsty.

didiman a person who works for the government and helps people to learn how to grow better crops or look after different kinds of animals.

diet 1 the mixture of foods that people eat. It is important to eat the right amount of food from the three food groups, which are growth foods such as protein, energy foods such as carbohydrates and protective foods such as fresh fruit and vegetables. This is called a balanced diet.
2 to control the type and amount of food that you eat.

digestive system the system of the body that breaks down food, beginning with the mouth and ending with the anus.

discrimination treating people differently or unfairly because of the place they are from or because of their gender, or because they are disabled.

draw a way of deciding which teams will play each other in a sports competition.

dribble to carefully move the ball forward little by little in a game of soccer or basketball.

duties the jobs or activities that people have to do or responsibilities that they must carry out.

economic the way that people earn and use money.

ejaculation the process in which semen is forced out of the penis. This usually happens during sexual intercourse.

election campaign the activities that supporters do in order to help a person to win an election.

environment the surroundings which may influence our growth, development and behaviour.

equality being fair, having the same rights as each other and the same amount of power in a relationship.

expectations the things that we should do or the ways that we should behave.

extended family a family consisting of children, their parents, grandparents and possibly uncles and aunts living closely together.

Fallopian tube (oviduct) the tube that carries eggs from the ovary to the uterus.

family planning deciding on the number of children that a couple want to have and the spacing between the births of those children. Contraception can be used in family planning.

fat one of three types of food that is needed in the diet.

fertilisation the joining together of a sperm and an egg cell. *See* conception.

fibre (roughage) the part of food that cannot be digested and absorbed to produce energy. Highly refined foods such as white rice, white sugar and white flour contain little fibre. Foods such as fruit and vegetables, nuts and brown rice contain a lot of fibre. People who have a lot of fibre in their diet do not usually have health problems such as constipation, being overweight or diabetes.

first past the post a way of deciding the winner in an election—the person who gets more votes than anybody else.

food chain the way in which some animals eat plants and some animals eat other animals, so that food is passed from one to another.

food poisoning an illness that affects the digestive system. Food poisoning is usually caused by eating food containing bacteria or poisonous chemicals.

freedoms the choices that everyone should be allowed to make.

gastroenteritis a sickness of the stomach and intestines. It is usually due to infection by viruses or bacteria or to food poisoning. It causes vomiting and diarrhoea.

gender being a girl or a boy, a man or a woman, which we learn from the community.
germs small living things that can make us sick.
grille a skin disease caused by a fungus that grows on the skin, often forming a pattern of circles or rings; also known as ringworm, tinea and sipoma.
gut feeling the feeling that we get inside our bodies that tells us that something is all right or is not all right.
haus tambaran a traditional house. The front of Parliament Haus in Port Moresby is built in the shape of a Sepik haus tambaran.
hazard a danger that is found in our surroundings.
health goals things that we try to achieve in order to be fit and well.
health promotion all the things that we do to prevent or reduce sickness.
HIV (human immunodeficiency virus) the virus that affects the immune system of the body and leads to AIDS.
identity individuality or personality.
immunisation a way of preventing sickness by giving a person an injection. Most immunisations are given to children, so parents must take their children to the clinic to get them immunised. Immunisations are recorded in a little book which the parents should keep in a safe place so that they know which sicknesses their children are protected against. *See* vaccination.
inequality something that is not fair or equal.
infant a child under one year of age. A child that cannot live without its mother.
inherited obtained from our parents.
injection forcing drugs or some other liquid into a part of the body by using a syringe.
instinct a skill or behaviour that people have without knowing or being able to explain why.
justice being fair and treating people equally.
kiap a patrol officer who carried out the work of the government in Papua New Guinea.
kula a trading relationship amongst people in the islands of Milne Bay Province in which shell necklaces are passed in one direction in a circle and armlets are passed in the opposite direction.
Leadership Code a set of rules for Members of Parliament and Senior Public Servants to follow.
leisure free time.
level of intimacy the closeness that people feel in a relationship.
lifestyle the way that people choose to live their lives, which varies from place to place and from time to time.
Limited Preferential Voting (LPV) a system of electing a person in which the candidate must receive an absolute majority, or more than half the votes counted, in order to win.
line umpire someone who helps the referee or umpire to decide if the ball has crossed the line in a game of sport.
locomotor skills the skills that we use when we move from place to place, like running, swimming.
long jump pit a hole in the ground that is filled with sand and used for the long jump and the high jump.
luluai a village elder or 'big man' in Papua New Guinea who was chosen to help carry out the work of the government in his village. *See* tultul.
malaria a disease caused by a germ called a protozoan which lives in the blood and is carried by some mosquitoes. People with malaria often have shivering, fever and sweating which can happen again and again; in some cases people can die. Malaria can be prevented by not being bitten or by taking chloroquine; it can also be treated with chloroquine or other drugs. There is more malaria on the coast than in the highlands of Papua New Guinea.
malnutrition not eating the amount and type of food that is needed to be healthy. This is very important when children are still growing.
menstruation *See* period.
microbe any living thing that is too small to be seen with the naked eye; for example bacteria, viruses and some fungi and protozoa.
mineral a substance found in food in small amounts that is important for good health.
mite a little animal that lives in the skin and causes itching.
modern societies people living a way of life which is typical for the present time and continues to change with the times.
nickname a name added to, or used in place of, a person's real name.
nicotine the drug found in tobacco and which is addictive. *See* addiction.
nominations choosing a person as a candidate in an election.

non-locomotor skills the skills that we use when we move but stay in the same place, like hitting a ball.
nourishing food that is healthy and satisfying.
nuclear family a family consisting of children and their parents living together.
nutrients the substances found in food which give energy and help us to grow and stay healthy.
nutrition 1 the food that people eat and the way that their bodies use that food. 2 the study of food.
obesity people who are very overweight are obese.
obligations the things that we are expected to do.
Ombudsman Commission an organisation set up by the government to deal with complaints against leaders. See also Leadership Code.
overweight being heavier than average for your height and age.
passive smoking breathing in the smoke which comes from the tobacco that other people are smoking.
peer pressure feeling that you have to behave in a particular way because other people of your age behave in that way.
penicillin an antibiotic that is made from a mould or fungus.
period when a girl or woman has a period, a small amount of blood and mucus flows from the uterus out of the vagina. Periods start when a girl is about 13 and continue about once a month until the age of 45-55, when they stop. This is a perfectly natural thing to happen and a woman having her period is not dirty and can do normal things. When a girl starts to have her periods it means that she can have a baby and when she is pregnant her periods stop; missing a period is often the first sign that a woman is pregnant.
pharmacist a person who works in an pharmacy and is allowed to give drugs to patients who have a prescription from a doctor.
physical the appearance or surroundings.
pollution waste produced by the activities of people that can affect the land, rivers, the sea and air.
polyandry when a woman has more than one husband. The woman may have children who have different fathers. Polyandry is one kind of polygamy.
polygamy when a man has more than one wife, or a woman has more than one husband, this is called polygamy. Polygamy is found in some parts of Papua New Guinea.
polygyny when a man has more than one wife. The man may have children with each of his wives. Each wife may live in her own house away from the other wives to prevent arguments. Polygyny is one kind of polygamy.
prescription a written instruction from a doctor to a pharmacist for preparing and providing drugs for a patient.
protein a type of food in the diet that, after being digested, is used in growth to form muscles, tissues and organs. Also known as growth food.
puberty the period of sexual development.
pubic area the area around the penis or vagina.
recreation things that we do to relax and enjoy ourselves. *See* leisure.
referee a person who controls a game of sport.
respect the way that we treat ourselves and others, laws and property.
responsibility 1 being trustworthy and able to answer for the way that you behave. 2 the job that a person has to do.
rights the things that people are allowed to have or do because of the law or because it is correct.
risk a behaviour that can have a bad effect on our health or well-being.
role the part that a person plays in a family, at school, in a sports team etc.
romantic love a dreamy kind of love in which both partners may see each other as ideal or perfect.
safety procedures things that we can do to deal with danger and keep ourselves safe.
scabies a disease caused by a little animal called a mite that burrows into the skin, causing bad itching.
scrotum the bag of skin that holds the testicles. The scrotum helps to keep the testicles at a lower temperature than the rest of the body, which is better for producing and storing sperm.
sculling gently moving the hands and arms to stay afloat in the water or move a little. *See* treading water.
semen the creamy liquid that contains sperm and that comes out of the penis during sexual intercourse.
sex 1 being a male or a female.
2 sexual contact between a man and a woman.
sexual development the changes that take place in our bodies as we develop from a girl to a woman and a boy into a man. *See also* puberty.

sexuality the way that we think, feel and behave because we are a male or a female.

sexually transmitted disease (STD) another term for sexually transmitted infection.

sexually transmitted infection (STI) also called sexually transmitted disease or venereal disease. Most STIs are caused by bacteria and many (though not all) can be cured by antibiotics if the person gets treatment early enough. AIDS, Donovanosis, gonorrhoea and syphilis are all STIs.

shoot to aim for the goal in a game of sport, for example, netball, soccer.

sign something that a health worker notices that shows that a person is sick, but which the person does not notice.

single parent family a family in which there is only a mother or a father to take care of the children.

spectators people watching a game of sport.

sperm the male sex cell. Sperm are usually found in semen and a single sperm fertilises the egg at the time of conception.

spleen an organ on the left-hand side of the body, below and behind the stomach.

sports injury any injury which occurs as a result of playing sport. Sports injuries often affect muscles, ligaments and tendons.

staple food the main food that people eat every day, like sweet potato, yam, banana.

stereotyping forming an opinion or making a judgment about somebody without having good reasons, especially when we think that a person has the characteristics of other members of the group.

strategy a plan to help achieve goals or objectives. *See also* tactics.

stretching exercises that people do before playing sport which help the muscles and joints.

submissive behaviour being quiet and passive.

subsistence agriculture growing and eating your own food; many people in Papua New Guinea do this.

suburbs the outer areas of a city.

survive to stay alive, to carry on.

symptoms something that a person notices which shows that the person is sick.

tactics the things that people do in order to achieve a particular purpose, like winning a game of sport. *See also* strategy.

tally room the place where votes are counted in an election.

testicles (balls) the two male sex organs which are held in the scrotum. The testicles produce sperm.

timekeeper a person who records the time taken, for example, during a game of sport.

tolerance accepting other people and their behaviour without being critical.

traditional societies people who still follow the customs and rules that were followed by their parents and grandparents.

travel move from place to place, for example, when playing sport.

treading water gently moving the legs and arms to stay afloat in the water. *See* sculling.

tuberculosis (TB) a disease caused by bacteria which usually affects the lungs and can cause people to have fever, spit blood and lose weight. People with TB can spread germs when they cough.

tultul a village elder or 'big man' in Papua New Guinea who was chosen to help carry out the work of the government in his village. *See* luluai.

typhoid a disease caused by bacteria that affects the intestines. It causes general weakness, red spots on the skin, chills and sweating. It is transmitted through food or drinking water that is contaminated with faeces or urine from an infected person. People usually recover naturally but the disease can be treated with antibiotics.

vaccination a way of protecting a person against a disease. A vaccine is usually given by injection, but can also be given by mouth and scratching the skin. *See* immunisation.

values the things that people say or think are important.

virus a very small microbe that lives on other organisms and so makes them sick. The common cold, influenza, measles, mumps, chickenpox and AIDS are caused by viruses. Many diseases caused by viruses can be controlled by vaccines, and drugs can be used to treat others.

vitamin a substance found in fresh fruit and vegetables in small amounts that is important for good health.

voters the people who are able to vote in an election.

wet dream semen which comes out of a boy's penis when he is asleep.